Keep Smiling!

CONFESSIONS
former
OF A COSMETIC DENTIST

DON'T EVEN THINK ABOUT AN EXTREME SMILE MAKEOVER UNTIL <u>AFTER</u> YOU READ THIS BOOK.

Copyright © 2010 CelebrityPress™ LLC

All rights reserved. No part of this book may be used or reproduced in any manner whatsoever without prior written consent of the author, except as provided by the United States of America copyright law.

Published by CelebrityPress™, Orlando, FL
A division of The Celebrity Branding Agency®

Celebrity Branding® is a registered trademark
Printed in the United States of America.

ISBN: 978-0-615-37083-5
LCCN: 2010927643

This publication is designed to provide accurate and authoritative information with regard to the subject matter covered. It is sold with the understanding that the publisher is not engaged in rendering legal, accounting, or other professional advice. If legal advice or other expert assistance is required, the services of a competent professional should be sought. The opinions expressed by the author in this book are not endorsed by CelebrityPress™ and are the sole responsibility of the author rendering the opinion.

Most CelebrityPress™ titles are available at special quantity discounts for bulk purchases for sales promotions, premiums, fundraising, and educational use. Special versions or book excerpts can also be created to fit specific needs.

For more information, please write:

CelebrityPress™,
520 N. Orlando Ave, #44,
Winter Park, FL 32789

or call 1.877.261.4930

Visit us online at www.CelebrityPressPublishing.com

CONFESSIONS
of a ~~former~~ COSMETIC DENTIST

DON'T EVEN THINK ABOUT AN EXTREME SMILE MAKEOVER UNTIL <u>AFTER</u> YOU READ THIS BOOK.

Table of Contents:

Introduction 9

Chapter 1
The 'Veneer Nazi' - Cosmetic Dentistry & The 'Veneer Nazi' 11

Chapter 2
Conspiracy Theories, OCD & SMILOREXIA 23

Chapter 3
Cosmetic Dentists and their Prey 45

Chapter 4
Tricks to Save Big Money at the Dentist 59

Chapter 5
Secrets Your Dentist Doesn't Want You To Know 71

Chapter 6
The Paradox of Conservative Cosmetic Dentistry 83

Chapter 7
Embarrassing Personal Experiences & More Insider Secrets 91

Chapter 8
Celebrities & Their Freaky Smiles 107

Chapter 9
Lies in Marketing & Primitive Dental Mutilations 125

Chapter 10
Gums, Your Kid's Ugly Smile & Avoiding Old-Fashioned Orthodontists:
Lets talk off the record 141

Chapter 11
It may be Chapter 11 for the 'Veneer Nazis' and a few Old Style Orthodontists unless they READ THIS SECTION: TOP SECRET BREAKTHROUGHS REVEALED ... 157

Introduction:

As a former cosmetic dentist, I speak to you in these pages as if you are a family member, perhaps a son or daughter halfway across the country, who is contemplating a new smile makeover. I am worried about what a cosmetic dentist might do to you and I am trying to steer you clear of danger. (For dental professionals who were attracted to the book, I'm just giving you my biased suggestions so you don't make the same mistakes I've made).

Due to the fear of reprisal, I can't expose individuals who continue to be "Veneer Nazis", but instead I'll share the reasons why I feel the cosmetic dental industry is itself in need of an 'Extreme Makeover'. We can't change what we've already done, but at least dental professionals caught up in the 'cosmetic tsunami' can make a fresh start from this point onward. The details I share are graphic, but someone has to speak for the defenceless teeth...I am the *Tooth Whisperer*.

If you think I am an alarmist, you may be right (but I am NOT concerned about the typical issues concerning mercury fillings, fluoride in your water, chemicals in white fillings, x-rays taken on pregnant women, what bugs may squeeze through the microscopic holes in the rubber gloves your dentist uses, or a few kids stoned on nitrous oxide being held down against their will for a mouth full of fillings). I have been horrified by the actions of "cosmetic fanatics" who have taken a useful procedure and applied it in the wrong places - as a cure for almost everything.

The dental association has known about this problem for years, but has been powerless to protect patients from it. Patients shouldn't avoid dental care, but they need to be aware of the dangers and myths within the cosmetic dental business. I have even become phobic of being called a cosmetic dentist, although patients would likely be confused if I advertised myself as an "Un-Cosmetic Dentist". The new conceptual type of dentist that I am promoting is very different, but one that I would recommend in a heartbeat over a 'Veneer Nazi'.

This is part of a personal crusade for public education about the abuse of patients' teeth at the hands of extremist cosmetic dentists ... but this is too big for just one rogue dentist who has gone A.W.O.L. Many dental professionals will secretly agree with the opinions included but most will not want to "cause trouble" for their colleagues so they remain silent. If the book changes how just one overly aggressive cosmetic dentist practices or stops one patient from doing something they shouldn't, many teeth may be saved. It's not about dentist-bashing (dentists on average are more intelligent, better looking and contribute more to humanity than the average person), it's about the freedom to warn the public that there is a problem.

A cosmetic dentist often becomes an unknowing host of a parasitic infection which affects how he/she thinks. As painful as it is, this book will attempt to 'dig the worm out from the flesh with a sharp stick, we will grab the parasite by the head and slowly pull it out of the dentist's brain'. Page by page, it will be agonizing for any 'diseased' dental professional to read (and enlightening for laypersons who know very little about this controversy), as the "cosmetic worm" is extracted, reeled, and twisted out on a twig. The industry that claims to make people's smiles more beautiful may in fact prove to be slippery and very ugly 'when fully exposed to the light'.

The most vocal critics of this book may in fact, be the ones with the most to lose, but let's look at the facts and see where they lead. For patients and dental professionals alike, this book may be shocking, infuriating, educating and hopefully sometimes entertaining. Don't mistake the fact that I like to amuse with the seriousness of this subject.

mz

Chapter 1
THE VENEER NAZI

Cosmetic Dentistry & The 'Veneer Nazi'

The field of aesthetic dentistry is a maze of slick marketing, financed by a billion dollar industry that is motivated by greed, and in many cases causes irreversible harm to its victims. Embarrassingly, the dental profession covers up a segment of practitioners that look you right in the face and try to convince you to do the wrong thing . Some of the worst offenders have climbed up the ranks of the cosmetic dental industry and warp dentists' perceptions about how to treat patients. . The wrong cosmetic dental treatment can look great on the outside, but can cause serious damage to your teeth. Unfortunately for the consumer, the profession keeps its 'dirty' secrets to itself to avoid the negative publicity.

"Cosmetic dentistry", even though it has the potential to do so much for people, has become a negative term to me. This book is not about 'good' cosmetic dentists, it is an insider's *exposé* of the little known hazards that are lurking within many unethical dental offices across North America. There are real risks to both your teeth and your pocketbook that you need to know about. This book will expose the significant dangers involved in *extreme smile makeovers* and other commonly advertised esthetic dental procedures, which are rarely revealed to the public. This book will also share new breakthroughs in cosmetic dentistry that could easily save you thousands of dollars, and help you avoid being treated by a 'Veneer Nazi'.

QUOTE: *"Washington woman, all diamonds and false eyelashes and big hair, but thin, like pictures of Auschwitz victims, ate nothing, waste of her own marvelous dinner, just pushed it around on her plate. Knobby collar-bones, claw hands and all those rings. Good solid bosom, surprising. Face getting all the help it could buy, skin taut under the tan. Kind eyes big white teeth. Capped. European women had crooked yellow teeth but at least you knew whose they were." – The Grown Ups.* Author: Victoria Glendinning {fiction}

Hurry...Cover your Mouth!

I don't want you to become self-conscious about your smile, but this is a warning: if you meet a 'Veneer Nazi' you are going to get picked to pieces. Cosmetic dentists are trained to notice things that 'even God' doesn't see. Small spaces, rotations and twisted teeth, uneven edges, the amount of tooth that shows when you smile, tiny enamel spots and mild redness in your gum line...these are all clues that you may have some shortcomings we are able to correct. What can you expect from someone who looks through magnifying glasses all day long?

Within micro-seconds we not only see your smile as imperfect, even hideous...undeserving of love...but cosmetic dentists are also appraising your ability to finance the comprehensive smile makeover. Listen, some of us even do a credit check on you before you set foot in our offices!

Did you drive up in a new Mercedes or a rusty old beater? The outside video surveillance already caught that one. Your shoes, are they Milano Blahnik as seen on Sex In The City or from PayLess? Your watch and accessories tell us what you like. Is your purse Louis Vuitton or just a Gucci?

Don't try to fool the fanatical cosmetic dentist with a cheap imitation or knock-off, or you'll be downgraded and have to settle for a generic 'take home' whitening kit, or, bite your knuckles...Whitening Strips (usually reserved for "Trailer Trash"...the kind of people who get the white suede leather waiting room chairs dirty, and yes, are always told at the front desk to try the office across town, where they take "that insurance").

This is what we do. And like a dog with an acute sense of smell, a cosmetic dentist is a different animal. Our eyes are more sensitive than most, perhaps at least equal to that of an artist who restores priceless paintings from the Old Masters at the Louvre, we are able to see subtle color and shade differences even within a flash of a nervous smile.

Our sense of smell is deadened by the fumes of all the glues we use to bond veneers…some of the bonding potions cost as much as $120,000.00 per gallon!!! Price is no object; after all YOU are paying for it. We "see" that you have bad breath long before we can smell it on you.

I admit most cosmetic dentists are twisted…with a smile fetish, so to speak. Looking at your teeth longingly like a vampire admires a neck, we can't wait to get closer. Your smile is as alluring to a cosmetic dentist as the enhanced cleavage of a Hooters® waitress for a newly released prison inmate. Parted lips make us crazy…and the worse your teeth are, the more we love it. Cosmetic dentists can be 'sick puppies'!

Our hearing is not great…the years of exposure to the high frequency sounds of the suction and high speed drill are to blame. We ask you about your concerns and your dreams, but we see much, much more wrong with you. We nod our heads and jot down notes, in spite of the fact we are barely hearing a word you are saying.

We judge you by your habits…if you smoke we will raise an eyebrow like a priest hearing about bestiality at confession, even though in our desk we may have an expensive box of Cubans. Drink red wine? You know how that can stain your teeth…the cosmetic dentist should know…the wine cellar is filled with the best vintages. Sweets are a definite "no-no" unless you have a dental degree. Double standards are something we have no qualms about…like a foreign diplomat, we claim special exemptions and immunity.

Our hands and sense of touch are exquisite…making a brain surgeon seem like a clumsy "sausage fingers". Houdini would have been an excellent cosmetic dentist. He would have enjoyed the magic we can deliver from 10:30AM to 2PM three days a week, less an hour and a half for lunch. We can sculpt like Michelangelo, and carve reality out of a lump of tooth-colored putty. Cosmetic dentists are gifted in certain ways and cursed in others.

As you turn your head looking for an escape path, we are already running through a systematic list of analyses, which will give us a solution to problems you never knew you had. I am now embarrassed by my obsession with smile imperfections and have consciously tried to shake much of the training, but I can't. Extreme cosmetic dentists can quickly get you out of almost any unsightly smile problem you possess, but often our cures can hurt you, and suck the cash right out of your line of credit.

TRUE/FALSE:
A Desperate Housewives TV star dated a Cosmetic Dentist?

Answer: As silly as it sounds, actress Teri Hatcher who plays Susan Mayer in the ABC hit series confessed on a major talk show (the one that keeps getting different time slots featuring "Big Jaw") that she had a crush on television's Extreme Makeover dentist Dr. Bill Dorfman. This led to a date after which Dr. Dorfman reportedly claimed in front of a huge dental audience that they "did it on the first date." Very likely he was just joking, and the crowd groaned in disbelief. Dr. Dorfman encouraged the cosmetic dentists in attendance to jump at the opportunity to duplicate the concept of the TV show in their own way, and the author confesses he did just that. A few years later, Dorfman, the successful LA cosmetic dentist and ZOOM Whitening entrepreneur married one of the contestants featured on THE APPRENTICE television program.

Rumor on the street is some of the people featured on Extreme Makeover have sued a few of the cosmetic dentists after the smile makeovers were completed. The exact details were unknown at the time of printing but it seems to relate to issues exposed in this book.

The Purpose of a Smile

In nature, animals make certain gestures and expressions as a way to interact and determine their social order. In prison, there are likely subtle clues the inmates use to warn each other that the guards are on their coffee breaks, and it's time to break in the new guy... who is alone in the shower.

Every man knows that a smiling woman is either intoxicated or a willing partner...there is no in between. Ladies learn to use their smiles very selectively if they know what's good for them. Women, on the other hand, know a smiling man is a dirty, filthy pig that is looking for trouble… or is at least good for a couple of free drinks.

Eons ago, friend or foe decisions had to be made in a fraction of a second to avoid being slammed in the skull with a rock. So, since Australopithecus strolled across the earth, and stopped for a quick drink at a real watering hole after a long day running from saber-toothed cats, the smile has evolved as a silent way to signal interest in the opposite sex or to just say "hello."

Due to the importance people put in their smiles, 'Veneer Nazis' have found ways to manipulate millions of dollars worth of unnecessary treatment out of the public. Much to the dismay of some of my peers, I'll share with you exactly how we've done it.

An Anthropologist seems to agree:

"Most men aren't picking up on the things we assume they're staring at," says renowned biological anthropologist Helen Fisher, PhD, author of *Why We Love* . The reason, she says, has a lot to do with evolution. "In general, men are wired to notice obvious signs that convey interest in mating — a warm smile, for example — and ignore other subtleties, like if your lipstick is faded," she explains.

NEVER Smile Back at a Gorilla

According to Reuters (2007): Gorilla jumps zoo fence and attacks

"Dutch Media widely reported that the woman misunderstood what she perceived as a smile from the gorilla. Experts suggest he was more likely to have been baring his teeth as a threat. Citizens lost sympathy for the woman after it emerged that she has visited the gorilla about four times a week and said that Bokito "remains her darling" despite suffering a broken arm and wrist and around 100 bites."

A Bad Cosmetic Dentist is like a Crocodile

A cosmetic dentist can be compared to one of those 18 foot crocodiles that you almost always see in a National Geographic television special on Africa. The wildebeests are thirsty after a long migration across the dusty savannah, and they crowd around a murky river with a steep bank...the ones on the edge are almost pushed in by those behind.

The cosmetic dentist has set up an irresistible lure...the promise of beauty, and you may be encouraged by your friends and family to "go first" to test the waters so to speak. Sometimes a boyfriend/girlfriend may be the one edging you forward towards the unknown.

Under the water a massive reptile is patiently waiting for the right moment. It just takes one of the land dwellers to satisfy the appetite of this big fellow. In a flash it is over, and the wild-eyed wildebeest is pulled into the water and disappears. And such is the interplay between a patient and an overly aggressive cosmetic dentist.

The crocodile is not going to waste time snapping at rodents or small birds. He couldn't be bothered, and uses the little 'feathered friends' to clean his teeth. A cosmetic dentist rarely bothers with the routine and small issues...'going for the kill' is the goal. Getting the big case...one or two big makeovers a month can easily allow the dentist to laze in the sun.

Being 'the croc in the stream' has been a bit of a monopoly, with few natural predators. Times are changing, and there is a new game in town that will be pushing the crocodile-like cosmetic dentist as we know it close to extinction, or force it at gunpoint to evolve into another more nimble animal...but this necessary change will occur only after the general public truly understands there are new alternatives that many cosmetic dentists don't want you to know about. Think of this book as a bridge across those dangerous waters.

<u>Hold off on any extreme smile makeover until you finish this book,</u> and you may see the world of cosmetic dentistry much differently. With any luck, you'll be healthier, wealthier, and more *naturally attractive* in the long run.

FACTOID: Some dental professionals admit that they inflate their prices for some "ethnic groups" that are known for their negotiating savvy. They will sometimes also substantially increase their fees and reduce the warranty if patients are rude and demanding.

Gallop Poll: Trust in the Dental Profession Drops

According to a recent subscribed dental report (Clinicians Report-

October 2009), over-promotion of aesthetic dentistry procedures has blurred the division between "need" dentistry and "want" dentistry. This has "confused patients and caused frequent incidents of overtreatment."

This report warns dentists "...during treatment planning, patients should be advised of the alternatives for treatment - **including the minimal ones**". After such discussion and patient agreement on the treatment, you have satisfied "informed consent" requirements."

It is very likely that while the highly respected authors of this particular newsletter attempt to "coach" dentists (who have strayed to the dark side of cosmetic dentistry) back to the side of respectability, a book such as this will have a more enlightening effect.

Kidnapping the Cosmetic Dentist's Kid

If Ashton Kutcher wanted to PUNK a 'Veneer Nazi' this is what he'd do. He'd set up a fake kidnapping of a cosmetic dentist's teenage son or daughter, and send an odd ransom request:

"*Dear Doc,*

I have your spoiled kid...and you have a choice to make. It could cost you nothing to get her back, but there's a catch...I am going to prepare all the kid's healthy teeth for porcelain veneers. For your information, I'm pretty good at doing them and actually used to be a member of a cosmetic dental organization. It's just I've gone a little wacko and want to veneer everyone! Alternatively you can pay me $50,000 and I won't do the veneer work. It's your choice. You have one hour to decide...we'll be in touch. And Doc...don't even think about calling the American Dental Association."

The typical dental professional exposed to this hypothetical situation - that could fit more comfortably into a SAW movie - would obviously be distraught, and very likely would be crying and screaming. However, once the dentist could think clearly, there is no doubt what the answer would be, and it wouldn't be the free teen porcelain veneer makeover!

Why EXPOSE the 'Dirt' on the Dental Profession?

Why would I, a simple small town dentist, (who by my own account, is only average at best with many failures that are humiliating to admit), want to become a whistle blower against certain members of my own profession? It could be related to childhood trauma, a car accident which may have damaged my ability to bite my cheek and maybe an umbilical cord twisted around my neck, but I wouldn't change a thing.

'Veneer Nazis' are epidemic; they've spread across North America and are now going for world domination. I probably should just keep quiet like the majority of the dental professionals and pretend everything is OK. This would help me avoid the backlash, but since nobody else is stepping up, here I am. I feel that more than a few dental professionals have pushed their luck and are taking advantage of people. Unfortunately, the dental profession is too 'wimpy' to warn the public about it. It's bad PR, and in this economy scaring off clients could put some good dentists out of business. In spite of all of this, I can't keep my mouth shut any longer.

I've paid a heavy price for my outspoken beliefs. Some colleagues have taken numerous steps, (sometimes resorting to actions which are likely borderline illegal or at least against fair trade practices), to stop me from exposing the truth. There are new developments that threaten their livelihood, but give patients additional choices between the extremes of 'quickie' porcelain veneers and traditional long-term braces with head gear.

Some have tried to spread negative rumors, but the latest research supports a new direction in cosmetic dental care. Since becoming disenchanted with being a traditional "cosmetic dentist", I've helped develop and promote the science that is now questioning many of the old outdated beliefs that were thought to be 'gospel'. Even after the myths are exposed, there is no way certain dental professionals will stop doing lucrative procedures which are grossly abusive - until the general public knows they are wrong and refuses to accept them.

Finally, I'm tired of listening to all the "bull crap" in the marketing from multi-million dollar companies that leads to misinformation for the consumer. I'm 'mad as hell and I'm spilling the beans' on all the stupid things that I've uncovered… this is only after decades of research and upper level training in the cosmetic dentistry from the best and the worst in the business.

NEGATIVE INSIDER REPORT TRANSLATED INTO COMMON ENGLISH:

The Myth of Instant Orthodontics: An Ethical Quandary

-JADA 139: 424-433, 2008 by Jacobson & Frank.

To paraphrase a recent dentist's article on Veneers: "Realignment/straightening of a healthy tooth using a porcelain veneer cannot be considered a minimal invasive procedure. Although speedier, it is doubtful the correction can be justified ethically. Three types of malalignment are recognized – rotation (twisted), labial and lingual displacement (pushed in or out of the best position) and spacing (gaps). For rotated teeth and ones that are out of position, the amount of drilling can range from none at all, to drilling deep into the tooth (sometimes into the nerve!). When spaces are closed with veneers the teeth look square and unnatural. The long term success of porcelain veneers is similar to full crowns. There are three forms of failure- fracture (67%), microleakage/decay/stain (22%), and debonding/falling off (11%). Therefore other alternatives should be considered." (ASK YOUR DENTIST ABOUT THIS!)

BRITISH DENTIST JOKE: I've heard there is a bad case of *"veneerial"* disease affecting many American dentists!

Dentists ONLY Show You What They Want You to See

Dental professionals need to balance "informed consent" with sales. Informed consent just means that you understand what you are getting yourself into. You know the risks of doing it, not doing it, what it will cost and you sign off on it. It doesn't allow the dentist to do a poor job, but it does warn you that not everything goes as planned. Lawyers simply say any complication is worth some cash, but the paperwork in the consent forms attempts to neutralize that argument. Things do go wrong even when the dentist is highly skilled, they just happen less frequently.

The problem is if you know too much about a procedure, it will often scare you off and leave the dentist with nothing to do. This is why you can't always expect the real facts from someone who is not going to 'make a dime' if you run away screaming.

I'm simply recommending that you learn what a good conservative cosmetic dentist would do for a loved one if he/she knew about the latest breakthroughs in aesthetic dentistry. There is a very good chance a "good" dentist will be comfortable with you knowing what is in this book.

WIKI-FACTOID: Professor Julius Sumner Miller (1909-1987), known to many as "The Professor" on TV shows including The Hilarious House of Frightenstein and The Mickey Mouse Club willed his body to the University of Southern California's School of Dentistry.

The Flamboyant Smile Detective

When you see a dentist, you hope the tooth doctor is going to help uncover problems before they become serious. In the case of the dentist who considers himself/herself a "cosmetic dentist", you may be getting more than you bargained for.

Not only are you getting a CSI investigation of a possible crime scene, you are getting a detailed smile analysis that is hyper-critical. You are at risk of being framed, and wrongfully accused of having an unattractive smile. Before this, you may have thought your smile was pretty nice, but if you make the mistake of answering "yes" to the question "Do you have any concerns about your smile?", you may be heading down a pathway that leads directly to your bank account. You should have remained silent.

I have been as guilty as anyone when it comes to this. Within a few seconds, almost before my eyes can focus, I pick out significant aberrations, variations slightly outside the average, and distractions usually missed by the casual observer. Like a laser beam, cosmetic dentists can zoom in on minuscule features and 'make a mountain out of a mole hill'. Dentists look for what is wrong and not what is right… that is also why many have a tough time getting along with each other. It is easy to second guess any professional's results and find flaws - while accepting a wider range of acceptability in one's own work.

Cosmetic dentists can take away your self-confidence. You may quickly lose your smile and start covering your mouth when you talk…all because of one of our 'picky' smile reviews. Unless you can anticipate this and steel yourself, you may become a victim of the subtle taunting and the undermining of your self-esteem..

Try this technique. If you start to get dragged into a big discussion about your smile that you feel is unfounded, just say "I never really worried about that, it's a bit of a family trait." That is a nice way of letting the cosmetic dentist know you are not going to be an easy sale. It may get the cosmetic dentist refocused onto a search for tooth decay, gum disease and signs of oral cancer or they may back off 'into the muddy waters' and wait for the next potential victim.

TRUE/FALSE:
Did Cosmetic Dentists get involved with a major player in the XXX Escort Business?

Answer: Some Cosmetic Dentists (including the author) actually learned marketing and business practices from a former big name in the High End Escort Business (translation: Prostitution). Google: 'Sydney Biddle Barrows' - for more information on this woman who now writes quite interesting marketing and customer service books. This gives new meaning to the term "Pimp Your Smile".

Chapter 2
CONSPIRACY THEORIES, OCD & SMILOREXIA

The Whitening Conspiracy

Smile whitening is the #1 cosmetic dental service that is requested in America. The problem is that there is a conspiracy between the whitening companies, the porcelain veneer companies, and the cosmetic dentists that you need to know about.

In this conspiracy theory, I propose that dentists and patients are being brainwashed into thinking that teeth need to be beyond natural white. The whiteness is beyond what most people can get with just whitening their teeth, and often is only possible with porcelain veneers. So first, patients do whitening, then they become addicted to the idea of whiter teeth. If the results are not what they expect, then they are sold on artificially white porcelain veneers.

It's almost embarrassing how artificial many of the porcelain veneer makeovers look these days. The teeth are all 'blinding' white and actually can make your eyes hurt if you stare at them too long. Cosmetic dentists and patients should 'get real', and back off from the idea that teeth need to be a color that is never seen in nature.

BIG TIP: Don't think your teeth need to be SUPER-WHITE

Celebrities in magazines have their teeth digitally whitened, and the lighting used in photo shoots often makes their teeth look much whiter than they really are. It doesn't hurt to have makeup and a tan either, since the contrast is what really makes white teeth "pop".

Tooth whitening is a great option and we will discuss it in more detail later, but I just wanted 'to hit you' with the concept early on that healthy teeth are slightly off-white, and not nearly as chalky white as many people imagine they should be.

WARNING: Beware of "Free trials" and online smile whitening offers. They are rarely free and consumers who thought they were signing up for a "free trial" of teeth whitening products are being repeatedly billed for services they didn't want, says the Better Business Bureau, which has been deluged with complaints around the country. Visit our website for more information.

Whitening Kiosks and why you get what you pay for

There is a new trend that's going on in almost every mall in North America. It's the economy whitening booths that claim to offer the same whitening power that a cosmetic dentist can. I agree that some cosmetic dentists overcharge for whitening, but there is no way anyone can compete with the whitening options that a dental professional can offer.

While in some areas the whitening booths have been shut down and judged to be illegal, many areas allow them to be staffed by people with little or no dental training. They sometimes get around the law by having the customer apply the whitening gel and then they set up the magic light.

They sometimes claim their light works better than the dentist's whitening light, but that's all hype. The light used by cosmetic dentists and these kiosks just causes a temporary whitening effect, due to the drying effect on the teeth - but really doesn't contribute to any long term whitening.

In short, I'd skip the economy kiosk and try to get a deal from a dentist. You shouldn't have to pay more than $350 for the one hour service, especially if you can encourage a friend to do it too on the same day. You can usually find someone with a special on whitening and if it's from a dentist it's almost guaranteed to be much better than the mall brands. As mentioned in the special reports on the website, there are a number of tips to get the most out of 'smile whitening', and one of them is brushing with toothpaste for sensitive teeth for a few weeks before whitening.

My bottom line is that you should talk to your dentist about whitening prior to doing a *smile makeover*. Sometimes things are more complicated, and for example you may have a dark tooth because it's dead which will need more than a superficial whitening treatment.

CRITIC'S COMMENTS:

I wouldn't call it a "conspiracy", as if the companies have colluded together to brainwash people. However, some companies do BENEFIT from patient's anxieties and fears of having "unhealthy & yellow" teeth, and take advantage of this trend. The goal of all businesses (at least those that want to be successful) is to supply their customers with a solution to a perceived problem. All cosmetic procedures, whether it's tooth straightening, whitening, tanning, acne-treatment, hair-coloring, Botox or breast enhancement, address our concerns about becoming ugly and old, and fulfill our desires to be beautiful and vibrant. The key, for us as healthcare practitioners, is to offer treatments that cause the LEAST harm (Hippocratic Oath) and the most benefit - the "biggest BANG for their buck". High-concentration whitening gels, often used in 1-hour procedures, can sometimes lead to bleaching & burning of the gum tissue (similar to how drops of Clorox bleach affect dark clothing). To avoid this, special materials and methods are used to prevent such things from happening. This is one of many reasons why any "power whitening" in-office treatment should be done by a licensed dental office, NOT the local mall kiosk-attendant. - Dr. Dwayne Kowalchuk, 2006 Valedictorian - Boston University School of Dentistry.

The GAP Obsession

I have made a small fortune over the years treating gaps between the teeth. Sometimes we move the teeth with braces, add bonding or even use porcelain veneers. The new trend that is threatening cosmetic dentistry is that people are noticing that gaps are often overlooked, and may even be the new "in" thing.

Tyson Beckford, from the Show "Make Me A Supermodel" may not smile very often, but as I recall, he has an eye-opening number of spaces that creates a knee-jerk reaction in the faces of most cosmetic dentists, who see them as a flaw. Other runway models are becoming recognized as unique and contrarian due to their gaps, and even the White House featured Condoleezza Rice and her noticeable space (diastema). As difficult as it is for me to admit, a gap between the teeth may not always be a big deal, and it may even look better than teeth that are too wide!

GAPTOID-1: If you are a woman with a gap between your teeth, and want to build self-confidence against pressures to fill it in or close it, buy the movie "Gap-Toothed Women" – http://www.lesblank.com/more/gap. (If male, simply rent the movie "Terminator").

GAPTOID-2: The Anti-Model is doing well in spite of a gap - visit the link http://runway.blogs.nytimes.com/2007/03/01/the-anti-model/

GAPTOID-3: How to tell if your gap is too big: Take a dime, sideways slip it between your front teeth...then try a nickel. If the nickel goes through then you are ugly...just 'joshing', there is no rule about gap beauty.

BASHED in the MOUTH?

If, like Tiger Woods, you occasionally get hit in the mouth, it is important to see a dentist right away. A number of simple things can be done by the dentist which may include re-implanting a tooth that was knocked out, re-positioning a tooth pushed out of position, repair of chips, and if a nerve exposure occurred you may feel better without the nerve. There are a complex series of decisions that need to be made but keep this in mind:

- If the tooth was knocked out, find it and either put it into your mouth or into cold milk and get to the dentist ASAP (...assuming you do not have life threatening complications that require going to the hospital instead).

- If you break a big chip of your tooth off cleanly, it can be bonded back into place if you can find it.

- DO NOT rush into the idea of getting chipped teeth veneered with porcelain, as repairs can be done easier with composite bonding, then for a few months the health of the nerve can be evaluated.

FACTOID: According to a recent study, coconut milk is a superior transport medium for a knocked out tooth (compared to milk, or water and some other thing you wouldn't have anyway). Time is the most important thing, if all you can do is spit in your hand and keep it moist on the way to the dentist, that's fine. (If your dentist is too busy look for an emergency dentist who can fit you in, look for the swollen faced cartoon in the Yellow Pages). Think about donating an easy-open can of coconut milk to your child's sports team.

If all that you have going for you are Your Teeth, then you're in TROUBLE!

While I agree your teeth should be clean and healthy, and your breath shouldn't make people wonder "who farted?", they don't have to be your finest asset. If your teeth are the only thing people notice about you then that says something, and it's not good. Cosmetic dentists are naturally fascinated by smiles because that's their business, but in the real world, teeth play a 'supporting role in your Broadway show' and should not be a distraction.

<u>If people are paying more attention to your teeth than they are to what you are saying, you either need a good cosmetic dentist or you have already had too much done to your teeth.</u>

The DDS=OCD

In many cases of obsessive-compulsive disorder the following conditions are observed:

- Things are repeatedly cleaned
- Items are lined up perfectly
- Something is repeatedly counted or doubled checked
- Items are not only lined up but they must be in a particular order
- A number of things are under complete control of the person with the disorder

- The person is susceptible to violent verbal outbursts or anxiety if others interfere with their rituals, or do not follow their way of thinking.

Dental professionals are systematically trained to become obsessed, in much the same way as many religious sects have rituals that give them a sense of well-being. OCD can be a conditioned or learned response, and can be easily spread among people who are in close proximity to each other, or are subordinates of someone with these compulsions. This has been observed in religion, gangs, extremist groups (KKK/Middle Eastern terrorist groups), political groups and even Boy Scouts.

Order and conformity becomes more important than critical thinking, and most of the ideas are accepted as "The Way". Once people get into a particular obsessive groove, it is extremely unpleasant for them to hear anything different, and therefore they tend to avoid moving into areas where they will be criticized for their beliefs. In the dental profession there are many polarized groups, each having their own OCD issues. As a patient, the single-mindedness of a particular dental professional can put your teeth at risk because the advice may be tainted.

As an example, if you asked an Italian which restaurant they would recommend, you'd likely be eating spaghetti that night. For a new smile, a typical cosmetic dentist will be serving porcelain veneers... extra white.

You KNOW your dentist is a little Cosmetically Obsessed when:

1. The doc uses more than one shade of composite filling material in your molars...yes, for the ones 'way in the back' that nobody sees.

2. He/she puts dark tints in the grooves to match the small cavities in the other teeth he/she is "watching" until they get bigger.

3. More time is spent taking pictures of his/her work than getting the filling done!

4. The doc charges twice as much for the "high cosmetic" fillings that really only make the photographs look better (and don't do a thing for your sex life). This obsession with a perfect match

may even make it more difficult for your next dentist to replace the filling. Using a whiter color than a perfect match may be better because unlike old silver amalgam, composite fillings are tougher to see during removal even with a microscope.

Don't be too Cocky…there's Nothing Better than your own Teeth!

There are some people who think they can neglect taking care of their teeth because they believe they can always get 'such-and-such' done (implants, dentures, crowns, veneers). They are making excuses for their bad habits, and they often find out the hard way <u>that even modern dentistry often falls short of the teeth you were given when you were sent 'out of the factory'</u>.

The best that dentists can do is come close to the amazing looks and function of your own teeth. They are little miracles of nature that have taken on shapes thanks to millions of years of evolution, or after some massive power made you and your teeth in his/her likeness. Either way, your teeth are designed to meet each other for chewing, or showing emotion to attract mates or repel them; when needed they can even bite off the ears or finger tips of those cavemen that don't get the hint.

Not everyone is born with what they think are perfect-looking teeth, but often they do not require nearly as much alternation as the cosmetic dentist will have you believe. With few exceptions, the more natural and untouched you can keep your teeth, the better off you will be. This means getting them repaired early and keeping the supporting gums and bone healthy too. Getting back to the basics will serve most people's needs better than overdoing it with aggressive procedures.

Implants are not a Perfect Replacement for your Teeth

Critiqued by Implant Inventor Dr. Gerald Niznick

The dental implant is a very important innovation which helps replace a missing tooth with a titanium "root". The implant requires good bone, good money, and a good dental practitioner to give it any hope.

Actually a single tooth implant replacement is less expensive than a 3 unit bridge, and the average life of a bridge is about 5 years whereas an implant may be a lifetime replacement. Therefore an implant is a better value that does not require cutting down good natural teeth adjacent to the empty space.

A patient cannot just get an implant and forget about it, he/she will have to take special care of it. Even with the best circumstances the dental implant is not nearly as perfect as a real tooth.

Absolutely wrong. The implant does not have a PDL so it is less susceptible to gum disease. It does not decay nor have a nerve that can die and require a root canal, which leads to the tooth becoming brittle and cracking. IT is better than a real tooth and has become the treatment of choice to replace a periodontally compromised, mobile tooth. Ask any Periodontist.

A real tooth has a suspension system and can take the little jiggling forces, while implants may not.

It is that jiggling force that encourages bone breakdown while an implant is like a pillar in concrete, and is therefore less susceptible to bone becoming loose, even in the presence of tarter build-up.

Your own teeth get hugged by the gums better and it is very difficult to put two implants together side by side and have them look right because the gums tend to flatten out.

Soft tissue sticks to the implant - in fact you do not even need attached gingiva. Yes, it is difficult to get esthetics of the papilla between two adjacent implants if you are placing them in an edentulous site, but if you do immediate replacement following extractions, you can easily retain the papilla.

If the implant is put in the wrong place you can't move it with orthodontic braces. If your gums shrink away from an implant then the silver-colored metal will be exposed. There is also a remote chance the metal in the implant could irritate your body in some way (while studies don't seem to suggest that as a problem).

So don't put the implant in the wrong position - today we have image-guided surgical procedures that allow you to place the implant on a computer screen using CT scan and then duplicate it in the mouth. In the esthetic zone if tissue recedes you will show metal, but today soft and hard tissue grafts, white zirconium abutments and proper surgical procedures can eliminate these problems. Remember, you are only using the implant were a tooth is lost so the question is not whether a tooth is better than an implant, it is how do you best replace a lost tooth.

Implants are also very expensive to offer because the parts, equipment and training cost a fortune. A company that has helped to bring prices down is called ImplantsDirect.com, which actually was founded by one of the pioneers of the dental implant. The prices from this company allow the dentist to pass on savings to the patient without any sacrifice in quality. As an example, the company makes an implant for about $22, and then they charge the dentist $150 instead of the $450 or so, which most implant companies charge. It was the only implant company that actually increased its business during the 2009 recession.

Thank you for the plug. Yes an implant costs about $22-26 each but that is only after investing $30M in the equipment and developing the products and only because we mass produce hundreds of thousands. There is the cost of advertising, customer support, sales, regulatory lawyers, accountants etc. For $150 we provide the implant, cover screw, healing collar, transfer and abutment. All the publicly held implant companies charge closer to $600 for all those components and with our all-in-one packaging, knowing what parts to order to complete the case is dramatically simplified because most times they are all included.

Even if Dr. Niznick and I do not agree on every issue, we both agree dental implants are an important addition to the field of dentistry. If you really need an implant, you need to find a very experienced dentist, periodontist, or oral surgeon, to help with the procedure, and often two are needed to get the job done. Some of the best courses are provided by specialists by the names of Dr. Carl Misch and Dr. Sasha Jovanovic, and dentists trained by these gurus have a better than average chance of doing an excellent job after they've had some practice.

So don't think you can just play hockey and kick box without proper protection… while smoking a pack a day, driving your car with a martini in hand without a seat belt, and ignoring your dentist's stupid little reminder cards - without having to find out the truth the hard way. Your own teeth are often the best thing you've got…you don't have to screw it up!

IMPLANT STORY:

"A patient of mine decided to go elsewhere for a dental implant, and ended up seeing a dentist who was rumored to have an alcohol addiction. After he had screwed in the implant and sat her up, the implant simply fell out! A year or so later, the dentist was forced into rehabilitation and has since retired. In short, be sure to see a competent implant surgeon, and hopefully one that is not near retirement." -mz

I confess…I'm GUILTY

I do not violate healthy teeth nearly to the same extent that I used to when I was a low level "Veneer Nazi ," but I still do things that I'm not proud to admit. I even get paid for it and often the patient is extremely happy. If patients knew what I know, they wouldn't let me or encourage me to do some of the procedures that I have done.

An attractive, newly divorced woman, was concerned about her slightly crooked front teeth. I didn't get her name from a list company specializing in the recently divorced, but I could have (supposedly a marketing company called MidWest Direct has 200,000+ names at any one moment and all you need to do is call 913-686-2220). I tried on at least two if not three visits to convince her to consider other alternatives instead of veneers, but she would not budge. I admit I could have tried harder and showed her things I am going to show you, but I didn't. I quit too early but at least she gave me an A+ for my persistence.

I numbed her up, grabbed my high speed drill and a big gold-colored diamond impregnated drill bit, and surveyed her smile. I hadn't done this for a quite a while since I pledged to not be a typical "cosmetic dentist", but I wanted to keep her as a patient. Her upper middle teeth were twisted, and I simply drilled away the amount of the tooth that stuck out too far. I drilled a little off the adjacent teeth (to be able to widen the middle ones a little), and then I drilled away some more tooth – to make room for the white filling material I was going to use for the veneering process.

There was so much drilling I was starting to get nervous about hitting the nerve. Sometimes we have to drill into the nerve, but generally, unless we plan it or warn the patient ahead of time, it makes us look dumb. I didn't mention anything about the possibility before I started, so it made me even more concerned as the drilling continued. My forehead got a little sweaty.

Finally I put down the drill, added my glues and layered on a white filling material called composite that would simulate a straight tooth. I knew it would be tough to match the color of the others since I was trying to do just two, but I thought I could get close.

I had to add some little tints to help match the white spots on her other teeth and then I covered them with a glaze, like a clear nail polish. They looked pretty good when I was done but I didn't take a picture of the "drilled-down" teeth because I didn't like what they looked like and didn't want to alarm the patient.

So I violated one of my own rules, which is to be as conservative as I possibly can, and if the patient doesn't want to listen to my advice, I should kick'em out rather than do something I don't think is in their best interests. But I, like hundreds of other dentists each day, did something that was according to my core beliefs… wrong. Well, maybe what I did was not "illegal", but it wasn't the best I could have done.

How do dentists slip into this pattern of doing something that they shouldn't? I can only speak for myself and speculate on the others. Sometimes it is greed, incompetence, laziness, budget concerns or stupidity on the dentist's part and /or the patient's. I think the more you know about what dentists have been doing the better.

PREDICTION: Veneer Nazis who have been very aggressive in their style of care will be moving outside the USA to avoid prosecution, unless they use specific techniques to protect their assets. After reading this book, many cosmetic dentists will start using much more detailed patient consent forms and fewer patients will be getting traditional "*extreme smile makeovers*"without first passing a written and oral test to prove they know what they are getting themselves into.

Twelve Simple Tips that can help you
Avoid Extensive Cosmetic Dentistry

1. <u>Routine Dental Care</u> - Catch problems early, treat gum disease and decay before it gets out of hand.

2. <u>Proper Home Care</u> - Actually brushing and flossing properly is important and so is using the correct toothpaste to match the risk factors you have.

3. <u>Wear a Seat Belt</u> - This saves pulling your teeth out of the dashboard.

4. <u>Sports Protection</u> - Wear a mouth guard and full shield protection with a helmet for high risk activities.

5. <u>Avoid Chewing Citrus Slices</u> - While Vitamin C is great for your oral health, chewing and sucking on lemon and orange slices excessively can dissolve the enamel off your from teeth and make veneers a necessity. Avoiding carbonated soft drinks and sports beverages also reduces your exposure to the acids that dissolve away your teeth.

6. <u>Assume babies and animals are going to whack you in the mouth</u> - Keep on your guard as 'the little rascals' are dangerous and can strike without warning.

7. <u>Don't walk with your hands in your pockets</u> - If you fall you need to be able to use your hands, not your face, to stop from hitting the pavement.

8. <u>If you grind your teeth in your sleep, purchase and wear a night guard appliance from your dentist</u> - People can save a fortune if they catch this problem early and simply wear the *bruxism* guard.

9. <u>Vomiting Disorders and Acid Reflux</u> - You really need to get professional help fast, see a medical doctor and a dentist for advice and visit AcidMouth.com.

10. <u>Avoid Illegal Drugs</u> - "Meth Mouth" is one of the ugliest things you'll ever see. Even legal drugs can have serious

side effects. Ask your pharmacist for the details, or visit our website for more information.

11. Don't get an Extreme Smile makeover if you don't really need one - Once you do it, you will be doing it again and again over your lifetime. We'll help you decide if you can be fine with conservative procedures and hopefully help you avoid an overly aggressive cosmetic dentist. If you've already been veneered from ear to ear try to delay replacing the veneers due to minor cosmetic issues.

12. If you get caught cheating on your spouse, hide the golf clubs.

Things the Dental Association doesn't want you to know…

The dental profession is very proud of its goal to eliminate tooth decay and gum disease, but if it did actually eliminate these problems, what would be left? Cosmetic dentistry! Making people look better is fine but the association is keeping a secret from the consumer. As a self-regulating profession, dentistry controls the licenses of its members and has the ability to control most of what a dentist can do and say. Unfortunately the public is at risk, because much of the focus is on how dentists "appear" to the public and not really on what they "do".

This PR campaign tends to hide the dirt within the profession, trying to sweep things quietly under the rug with very little 'fanfare'. When a celebrity goes into rehab, the tabloids are all over it. When a dentist strays out of line, they are usually punished behind closed doors. You would not believe the 'nut cases' that are in our profession…besides me.

This special treatment of our idiosyncrasies respects the massive investment in the dental professional, who basically is a person who can only do one thing…fix teeth. After years of training there were many opportunities to weed out the ones that shouldn't be there, but generally if you get the grades you can get through the system. The 'extreme' cosmetic dentists, who in my opinion have become dangerous to the public, are loosely regulated by the associations and get away with things they'd never be allowed to do in dental school.

You will rarely hear about cosmetic dentist violators, I suspect partly because the association is supported by many of the companies benefiting from the misuse of cosmetic dental procedures. They are a giant Multi-Billion dollar lobby group. This conspiracy manipulates the dental profession and is putting your family's smiles at risk.

The 12 things you can't rely on to help pick the Perfect Dentist

To find the right dentist you can't rely on any of the following:

1. He/she attends the same church.
2. Teaches at a university.
3. Is a member of a particular dental organization or is a specialist.
4. Advertises more hours of education than required.
5. Has years of experience.
6. Is fresh out of dental school, supposedly with the latest ideas.
7. He is wealthy, or appears successful.
8. By sex, race, or sexual orientation.
9. Recommended by a friend.
10. Seems nice and friendly.
11. The dentist is in good-standing with the college.
12. The dentist has the coolest ads or is a "celebrity dentist".

Unfortunately there is nothing I can say to help you find the dentist of your dreams. Most are good, half are above average and half are below average in skills. The ones I want you to worry about may be technically excellent at what they do, but they may do things that may not always be in the best interests of your teeth. All you can do is educate yourself and not fall for high pressure sales techniques and marketing that hide the truth.

Sometimes it's YOUR Fault

There are a few patients who are just 'way too picky'! Some are obsessive-compulsive types who tend to zero in on the most microscopic imperfections. They are rarely pleased with the color, shape, or position of their teeth. They were meant to be orthodontists or cosmetic dental board examiners…but they missed their calling.

As mentioned, the cost of these desires for perfection, whether from the dentist's side or the patient's will be very high. Time, money and higher risks of complications will follow the multiple attempts to reach any goals set at stratospheric levels.

Frankly, these types of patients are a real 'pain in the butt' to treat (at least for me), so they deserve to find a practitioner who is equally fussy. If you like name calling, they can be called *"Smilorexics"* for their obsessions about their smiles.

Going to the Dentist is pretty Safe UNLESS You Want a *Smile Makeover*

Years ago, there were fears dentists would intentionally inflict people with the HIV virus, then there was the mercury filling scare, the 'pervert' dentists, and the 'white filling' issue. Now, an even bigger problem has been the 'makeover' craze. On average, dentists in modern countries are pretty competent. While some are more artistic than others, the function of their work is usually acceptable. If someone has a problem with a dentist, they can go half way down the street and find another one.

My warning for you is about cosmetic dentists trained in a certain form of "aggressive" *smile makeover* treatment. Dental school didn't discuss the concept at all when I was a student, but once a dentist has graduated, there are courses that teach a style of aesthetic treatment that can be very harmful. These dentists look and talk like anyone else, but there are subtle differences - which I'll try to share with you to help you recognize the signs of trouble.

I want to get my point across, so this book avoids most of the technical jargon that dentists tend to use when talking to each other. I dumb things down naturally. If another dentist wants to debate this issue with me they can try, but I'd take any dentist to task who disagrees with my feeling that more than a few patients are being over-treated in the name of cosmetic dentistry.

If you are looking for a dentist specifically for a *smile makeover*, I'll advise you right this second… 'pour some cold water on yourself' and read on. Whenever you are buying anything expensive, or making an irreversible decision, and a *smile makeover* is usually irreversible, <u>you must take your time and do your research carefully</u>.

Hot or Not?

If you don't think your smile is attractive, you now don't even have to leave your home to get some personalized advice. There is a cutting edge new website that rates your smile and offers constructive suggestions from some of the world's top smile experts.

You simply log onto the site www.*RateYourSmile.com* and post photographs of your face and smile. There are some particular pictures that should be included as follows (they are clearly demonstrated on the site):

1. A picture of your whole face with your biggest natural smile. This helps the team analyze the relationship of your facial features and lips to your teeth. This facial analysis is very important to determine if you are a candidate for simple orthodontics, bonding, or something more complex like skeletal surgery.

2. A close-up of your smile. In this picture you should pull your lips back with your fingers, and open enough so your lower teeth show too. Be sure the focus and flash capture the fine details.

3. A Profile (side view) photograph will provide information related to your skull and jaw size relationships. Do not stick your chin out on purpose or you may be told you look like Jay Leno.

4. Additional photos, plus a picture of any x-rays like the full mouth "PAN", would be great.

You could also load a link to a You Tube video which captures the images mentioned above. A sample on the website helps you get the most out of this new program - which allows access to clients across the world.

Dental experts will then use the information you provide to give you some suggestions that you can consider. On occasion, people fuss over something that is quite a natural or even a desirable feature. It is often a matter of preference and personal opinion.

The smile experts come from various backgrounds and can often disagree with what is best in a particular situation. This reflects the reality of any aesthetic consultation, where there simply is not just one right answer. Some suggestions will be more conservative and more affordable, while others may be at the other end of the scale.

These online services at **RateYourSmile.com** are not a substitute for an actual visit to a dental professional. A dental professional can chat with you, look in your mouth, review your original x-rays (radiographs), and check your oral health and jaw joint (TMJ) condition. However, this new option may give you a fresh perspective that could save you money.

The Playboy Study

During one of my UCLA training sessions in cosmetic dentistry in Los Angeles, I saw an ad in the paper that was promoting a Playboy Playmate reunion. Many of the Bunnies from the beginning of the magazine were going to be there, plus a few celebrities including Gene Simmons from KISS, so I looked at this as a potential learning experience.

KISS was a bit of a crutch for me during my ugly teen years, and the chance to meet one of the founding members was huge and an obvious excuse to see a few Playboy Bunnies. I skipped out on part of the class and grabbed a taxi to the convention center. It was after buying the ticket at the door that I had found out that I had already missed the chance to meet Gene Simmons; his appearance was the day prior. I had to settle for a 'maze' of playmates.

The whole place was set up so you could stroll and meet these special women who bared more than their souls for a 'brief-less' appearance in one of the most successful magazines in history. While I was not a subscriber, I have to confess that I had only purchased one of the magazines in my whole lifetime (a girl I knew had a picture in that issue).

The real reason for attending was scientific... I was looking at this visit to the Playboy Reunion as an opportunity to do a study of Playboy Bunny smiles, to see if they were that much better than the smiles of "normal" women. This would be ground breaking, and I thought it possibly could serve as material for an article in a dental journal.

I wanted to know if these women were somehow more gifted in the smile department...were their teeth especially perfect to make men from all around the world want to buy pictures of them, without the distraction of clothing. As a cosmetic dentist, I had a belief that they somehow had super-smiles. As I went from table to table, I looked at the pictures of their magazine spreads and said a few bashful "hellos". I regret now being too cheap to purchase the commemorative album which I could have had autographed by the girls for only $10 per playmate. Fortunately, I did have my camera and after explaining my clinical study of Bunny smiles, a few of them let me take close-ups of their teeth.

It didn't take long for me to realize that most of the Bunnies, who ranged from young women to grandmothers (the convention featured women featured over the whole history of the Hefner business), had nice smiles but they weren't exactly perfect by the standards we were being taught. I decided to take a step back and look at these people more from a layman's point of view. At first everything was blurry... my intense focus on their enamel was like looking at a book too closely and then having to look up. I rubbed my eyes and suddenly they came into focus...WOW!!! I had been missing out.

Now I could see the big picture, and all those mathematical calculations of tooth proportion, amount of gum showing in a full smile, and midline measurements didn't seem to matter at all. I patiently waited in line for the more popular playmates, and spent a few moments posing for pictures with them. I had just enough film and battery life to be able to record some of this experience for eternity, Gene Simmons or no GS.

There were a couple girls that simply exuded a raw magnetism. It wasn't their teeth at all...although if they didn't have teeth they would be somewhat less attractive - it was their whole being that overcame us. We babbled and smiled and occasionally got hugs from these bombshells that were more than just a nice set of teeth. One Ukrainian girl who said she lived in NYC was particularly attractive, and her curves (which I would have easily missed if I wore dental magnifiers), gave me a mental lobotomy...I wanted to become a groupie.

Perhaps I should have put my dentist glasses back on, but I instead soaked up her essence and squeezed a few pictures of us together. Unfortunately, I was later to be gravely disappointed when I found pictures of her were out of focus and did nothing to capture the true spirit of the moment. Some lucky man is now spending every penny he has to make her happy and it would be all worth it.

One picture that did turn out clearly was my time with the Playmate of the Year. She sat on my lap, and my face filled with joy as I saw things up close that most boys and men had to settle for on printed paper. We exchanged pleasantries and I told her I hoped she would become very wealthy in the future. She liked that and wished me the same. Somehow I knew it would be much easier for her than me, but I was not jealous, I was just happy to be alive with a new set of eyes. 'To hell with being a cosmetic dentist…I wanted to see the real world!'

FACTOID: Even though the UCLA Aesthetic Dental training program was cutting edge at the time of the events shared above (1999), only about 1% of the curriculum was dedicated to discussing treatment described in this book. It missed out on simple steps now considered by many including the author as essential in a *conservative smile makeover*. A submission was made to Dr. Brian LeSage, Program Director, to include new developments that are revealed in this book, but the offer was declined.

No-Drill Veneers?

A savvy marketing company came up with the idea to promote a type of porcelain veneer as a way to make people look better - without drilling down their teeth or using a needle to freeze them first. A very simple procedure for the dentist and very easy money… that's always a good way to get a cosmetic dentist interested. It went straight to the consumer and promoted "drill-less" veneers which was an embarrassment to the cosmetic dentists who were not thrilled with the alternative, but it forced many to take the course to meet the demand from the public.

The brand you will recognize from television ads and brochures at the dental offices that offer it, but for legal reasons we'll just say it is a brand of veneers that rhymes with "Lube Your Gears". The basic idea is to cover the front teeth with a thin layer of porcelain to make them whiter, straighter and sometimes longer. They are expensive relative to the amount of effort that is needed, and if a tooth is out of alignment some drilling may be needed.

From what I've seen most people end up with an artificial looking smile, perhaps due to the opaque white shade that seems to be popular. Their teeth are a little thicker due to the layer of porcelain and adhesive - which glues them securely to the teeth. While they are fast and easy, you could often get a more natural-looking improvement with professional tooth whitening and selective use of composite bonding and reshaping…a much more affordable solution with very good results.

Some traditional cosmetic dentists look down on this type of veneer as a "veneer for beginners", but there may be certain situations where a "no drill" veneer may be a good idea. As an example, small teeth that are spaced may be easily improved with this technique, but you'll have to ask your dentist if it would be right for you.

CRITIC'S COMMENTS:

"No-preparation veneers have their place, but they are MASSIVELY overused. Spin and hype makes patients believe that traditional veneers are no good and that somehow no-preparation veneers look as good and are stronger. The truth is that no-preparation veneers have margins that are difficult to hide, so they stain more easily. I bet they didn't tell you that in their advertising! Any dentist is capable of placing no-preparation veneers. Any lab technician is capable of making no-preparation veneers. And yet the world's best dentists and technicians rarely make them, because they prefer quality and longevity. Don't get me wrong, I occasionally place them but they are overused and can be dangerous in giving patients high expectations and low end results." – Dr. Pav Khaira, www.RedSkyDentalSpa.com

Cosmetic Dentists Try to Steal Each Other's Patients

In these competitive times, dentists try their best to keep their own patients while also trying to solicit patients from other offices. It's a 'dog-eat-dog' world, and your teeth are valuable not only to you, but to the dental professionals in your area. I 'feel out' patients who I may see as an emergency, to see if they want to come back to my office instead of going back to their "old dentist". I wouldn't be asking if I felt they were not my type, but if I saw something really worthwhile that I could do for them, it is tough to control the urge to steal them.

Patients can be swayed by bribery, specials, bad service at their previous office, better hours, shorter waiting times, cleaner offices, closer locations and nicer staff and dentists. Televisions on the ceiling help too.

If I knew the patient was seeing a dentist who was not doing what I thought was best for them, I would 'work my magic' and attempt to "wow" them with some interesting option that they may not have heard of. For example, if they had a broken tooth and their dentist never mentioned the importance of the occasional crown/cap/onlay to prevent a tooth from cracking, they would get a special presentation.

If by chance the patient had a quote on some of their treatment and were in for a second opinion, it was pretty easy to find a way to give them a better deal - or come up with an alternative that would offer them something to consider. It wouldn't be very smart to suggest something that was more expensive, painful or life threatening.

If one dentist can do something better than their competition, then I think they should have the right to make a bid for your business. That's how the world is supposed to work, but the dental profession wants to pretend we're all buddies. We're not. The dental profession is a huge collection of little cliques that pretend to get along.

Chapter 3
COSMETIC DENTISTS AND THEIR PREY

The Perks of being a Cosmetic Dentist

When I told a sage old retired school teacher friend about my plans to go into the dental profession, she smiled, showing her worn denture teeth. Then she said "Oh! You'll be a meal ticket". At the time I didn't understand what she meant... now I do.

Cosmetic dentists can generate an upper middle class lifestyle and easily have many of the things usually associated with movie stars and successful rappers. In my case, as a modestly successful cosmetic dentist I have had a collection of high end sports cars including a Porsche 356 replica, a red 1965 Corvette, a Dodge Viper GTS, a brand new Lamborghini Gallardo. Not all at the same time like Jay Leno (and I don't think Jay leases his cars), but one at a time, with modest retreats into Volvo and Toyota.

My old motto was: when a woman you've never met swings a bra out her vehicle window at you, you know you've made the right car buying decision!

Cosmetic dentistry can support a luxurious lifestyle, but it should not be at the expense of mistreating patients. There are ways to be successful as a dentist without being out of control, and dentists with an open mind will find new ways to have their toys, doing what I think is more conservative treatment for their patients. Dental professionals should make much, much more than the average person who does not run his/her own business (dentistry is tough, stressful work), and dentists need to be better salespeople...they just need to sell what is right for the patient.

HOT X-Ray TIP for ADULTS:

If you have white fillings or a higher than average risk of tooth decay or gum disease, ask your dentist to take four "bitewing" x-rays at every other check-up, because when they only take two they often miss critical areas. In addition to this, a second x-ray will confirm a cavity which sometimes either is tough to see or was a ghost image on the film (not a real cavity). By catching a cavity early, the small additional cost of the extra x-rays will be saved many times over by avoiding expensive complications. Doubling the number of x-rays does <u>not</u> double the cost, and can actually save you money in the long run.

Do you suffer from the "Over-Done" Syndrome?

Some people just try too hard. Even if you know that you have this problem it may be tough to break out of it...some people mistakenly think more of something is better. Which of following apply to you?

- You are platinum blonde (with dark roots)
- Crave lots of attention
- Highlights in the hair
- Clip-on hair additions
- Long fingernails painted in wild colors
- Push-up bra or breast implants
- Heavy make-up that seems to get thicker each year
- Fake eyelashes
- Colored contact lenses
- Daily visits to the suntan studio even on sunny days
- Botox injections a few times a year

- Recent plastic surgery or liposuction
- Eyebrows tweezed
- High heels
- Pedicure addict
- Excessive jewelry
- Very tight clothing
- Low cut jeans and tops-you have cleavage visible from the front and the back!
- Obsessive about having whiter teeth than everyone else.

If you said "yes" to two or more of these, and you are male then you may be a transvestite. If you are a woman and not a talk show host with the first name Ellen or Rosie, then you probably do not need to do the quiz…as you almost certainly suffer from this disorder. By trying too hard to look good you may end up being less attractive than you should be. A simple rule to keep you out of trouble is try to do more with less.

Getting your teeth overdone cosmetically is as out of style as a mullet or a comb over, and the obsession will cost you money, time and increase the risk that you will end up losing your teeth.

The "Natural" Look is always in VOGUE

Teeth are not an accessory that should be changed with seasonal fashion trends. They are alive and extensions of your body that have a character all their own. As long as your teeth are not distracting in a negative way, they may be just fine.

Even the top fashion experts and designers have teeth that are less than ideal. (Take Karl Lagerfeld as an example, if you peek in his mouth you'll find an assortment of mismatched porcelain crowns that have more assorted colors than most spring clothing collections.) It may be more affordable and safer for you to invest in stunning or unique designer clothing and designer eyewear, than it is to mess with your smile. Coming from a former cosmetic dentist this may be surprising, but it's my absolute opinion that it is always best to go for the natural look.

Spaces or a little crowding in the teeth can be considered French couture. Just say "no" to fake-looking teeth and you'll be much better off in the long run. If the top staff at Vogue can get away with normal looking teeth, then so can you.

Make Me Beautiful Doctor!

A cosmetic dentist has a huge responsibility...being the person who is counted on to make one of the bodies largest and most visible orifices more attractive. The other openings have much less pressure.

Sure your eyes can get lifted with surgery, colored with contacts, enhanced with eyelash treatments, and surrounded with eyeliner and makeup. You can dress them up with exotic eyewear. Your ear orifices and nostrils are less important, and piercings and jewellery serve as a distraction for these pairs of holes.

The mouth, on the other hand, can be enhanced with a ridiculous amount of modification, which seems out of proportion to its relative size. As discussed in the cultural section, oral modification is nothing new, but the investment which is demanded by cosmetic dentists for such purposes may exceed its value.

While the woman who spent over $1,000,000 on plastic surgery to look like a Barbie doll may get free publicity, her stupidity and obvious obsessive disorder were grossly abused by the surgeons. I have to admit I am also guilty of such abuses of people's irrational desires, since many people who come in for cosmetic treatment already are nearly perfect...but 'a guy's gotta make a living, right?'

Even at the peak of my cosmetic dentistry career, I resisted trying to sell the "big ticket" makeovers. In my mind I could not justify the fees. You could send your child to Harvard for a year for the same price of a 'moderately priced' full- porcelain makeover. Is it really worth that kind of cash?

On a per tooth cost basis, the makeover quickly adds up, but the amount of time it takes to drill down a group of teeth is not that much more than doing one. There rarely is a volume discount unless the cosmetic dentists are starting to set up in Costco. Frankly, knowing what I know from being on both the cosmetic dental side and the anti-veneer side, it would be better to pay to have less dentistry done.

<u>A good cosmetic dentist, who is not under the spell of a recent porcelain veneer makeover course, would probably rather throw him/herself in front of a bus instead of having one of their teen/adult kids undergo a porcelain makeover to correct crooked, but otherwise healthy teeth. Think about it!</u>

I know after I completed a number of cosmetic dentistry courses, I was tempted to have my teeth straightened with porcelain veneers, but I'm very glad I postponed that idea. I do regret some of the makeovers I did as a cosmetic dentist, but that is simply 'enamel down the drain' now.

FACTOID: New dentists often try to add grey hair color to fool you into thinking they are more experienced, and older dentists often color their hair to hide the fact that they may be "less hip" than they want to appear.

Why HD Television may Save your Smile

Once you get an HD television hooked up to your dish or cable system you will see things you've never seen before…human imperfections. Actors and actresses…newscasters…they often have bad skin (even Brad Pitt has a few pock marks), and less than perfect teeth. This may help break you of the false belief that somehow everyone on TV is perfect, and if they weren't, they wouldn't be rich and famous.

The truth is many of the leading men and women will not be as flawless as you originally believed. Hopefully you'll be a little less hard on yourself regarding how your teeth appear to others. By breaking the obsession with perfect teeth, you may avoid being over-treated by a cosmetic dentist - who is all too willing to give you a makeover.

Crazy XXX Stories from Dental Assistants

It's pretty funny to listen to some of the stories from dental support staff. One assistant told me she worked with a very religious dentist, who happened to be treating a patient with the help of nitrous oxide. Laughing gas can give people a floating or calming sensation or it can make them smile and not really care. In other circumstances, it can cause sexual arousal and in this story, the female patient forgot where she was and she began to fondle herself right in the dental chair in front of the dentist and the dental assistant.

The dentist immediately jumped off his dental stool and left the room, while the assistant turned down the gas and reminded the patient where she was, and tried to explain what was going on. This is a side effect that we usually don't advertise or discuss, even though it could be 'good for business'.

The same dental assistant had worked for another dentist who was actually addicted to nitrous oxide and spent noon hours breathing the "happy air". His fairly open habit was justified by him as "taking the edge off" of his work stress.

FACTOID: Dental Assistant to Playboy Bunny - **Kendra Wilkinson** This reality star and ex-girlfriend of the infamous Hugh Hefner hasn't always been pure glitz and glamour. Wilkinson was working as a dental assistant in San Diego when Hefner came across a photograph of her that had been sent to his mansion. Wilkinson has said: "(Before meeting Hef,) I was living day by day, working as a dental assistant, living on Easy Mac and Spaghetti O's,"

The Scary Thing is ALL Cosmetic Dentists think they are helping you

As an extension of the health care system, dentists are trained to be healers, and never want to cause you harm. Cosmetic dentists, and probably even most 'Veneer Nazis', want to make you look better, and most have good intentions, but that is not enough.

Just because a professional really believes in the recommendations or treatment doesn't mean you should get it done. *Many cosmetic dentists have veneering stamped in their mind as a 'miracle cure'. It is not.*

When someone really believes in his or her treatment a patient is much more likely to follow their recommendations. This over-confidence is scary to me now, because so much of what has been taught to cosmetic dentists now is obsolete, and getting thousands of dentists to give up a dependence on a proven money maker will take years.

One of the goals of this book is to not only educate readers about new innovations, but it is to 'spook' the "veneer or die" cosmetic dentists that have ventured onto the 'dark' side and warn them that the game is up. Veneers can be fantastic when used appropriately, but some dentists use the procedure without careful consideration of more recent alternatives.

TRUE/FALSE:
All teeth that get root canal therapy MUST be crowned to prevent them from breaking.

Answer: It's a myth that every tooth that gets root canal therapy should be crowned/capped. If the tooth is a front tooth (one of the top front six teeth or lower front eight teeth), AND if it is still mostly intact structurally then studies show it can often do very well without extra treatment. Our website may go into more detail about other considerations a dentist may discuss with you.

Doing the WRONG Thing Really, Really Well

Extreme cosmetic dentists are probably the most perfect examples of my theory of "doing the wrong thing, really well...sorry I don't want to be too insulting ...I mean really, really well". The best of the best are so picky they will fuss over microscopic things that not even your closest friend or most intimate lover would ever notice in a lifetime. These cosmetic dental people are good at what they do...I, along with many respected authorities in the dental field whose names would not mean anything to a patient, just disagree with it.

If cosmetic dentists are doing a smile makeover they analyze all your faults, plan your new smile, sell you on the idea, and after you give them permission they get to work. They will spare no expense to make sure you have the most technically perfect smile in the universe 'according to their rule book'. It will be right out of a cosmetic textbook: the color, the gum line, the size and shape of each individual tooth, will be perfectly symmetrical and mathematically correct...but it may still be all wrong.

It's wrong because their work will be <u>'too damn perfect' and wrong because they often damage the teeth in the process</u>. A denture looks perfect, but real teeth aren't. Nature is not perfect...*star flakes* as an example are all a little different, and teeth all should be a little different too.

Often in an attempt to try to get things "just right" a cosmetic dentist will do the porcelain veneers over and over again. <u>If you let your cosmetic dentist repeatedly cut off your veneers in an attempt to get things "perfect", this is very harmful to your teeth</u>. 'Get your ass' out of the dentist's office and don't worry one bit if he fails his/her fancy cosmetic dentistry accreditation examination.

Beware of the "Fly & Fix" Cosmetic Specialist

If you travel by commercial airliner, you will eventually be tempted to open one of those sticky in-flight magazines. The real danger is that you'll open the magazine and become enthralled with the glitzy ads from the cosmetic dentists that want you to fly in for an *extreme smile makeover*. I seriously looked at this concept too…at least in the days where I was primed up and partially under the spell of being a rock star cosmetic dentist. The hope with this type of targeted ad is the dentist will find a wealthy client (poor people don't fly…they're lucky just to ride the bus on special occasions). The rich like to be pampered and enjoy the limo ride to the office and the promise of fast and top level service.

The fact is, these cosmetic professionals are very focused on closing a sale on a "big case" or extreme makeover using porcelain veneers. Regardless of the fact that many of the clients could likely be saved thousands of dollars through more conservative alternatives, the veneer is the treatment of choice for fly-in makeover offices.

Other alternatives are much more difficult to provide in a "hit & run" type of service. While the before and after pictures may be enticing, if you truly need cosmetic dental care, you will likely be better off finding a professional who practices near you.

Are Some COSMETIC DENTISTS DANGEROUS???

Actually, a few cosmetic dentists and all of the extremist 'Veneer Nazis' are probably (off the record, I'd drop the 'probably') causing more harm than good. The fact is many leading dental educators are issuing powerful *warnings within the profession* (not publicly) about this specific problem. The violators can be at the start of their cosmetic training after a weekend course, or they may be considered pillars of the profession. The higher a dentist climbs in cosmetic dentistry organizations, the greater the pressures to strive for ideals thought to be part of a perfect smile. The examiners literally put your work under a microscope and pick a dentist's work down to the smallest detail. If the cosmetic dentist does not have OCD when he/she starts their quest to be "accredited" in a cosmetic dentistry club, they certainly will end up that way. 'Veneer Nazis' are not born, they are brainwashed with years of exposure to party propaganda.

While at first having the ideal smile may seem to be a good thing, the "perfect smile" is a concept that can be both costly and harmful to patients. The cosmetic dentist sometimes treats natural variations like a cancer. Many mild imperfections in a smile get very little notice from people in the real world.

To explain how certain ideals create more cost to you (the patient), consider this:

- If you have the "wrong color" of enamel it could mean whitening or veneering. Cosmetic dentists likely will not tell you what a natural color is, but instead share with you how white you could get your teeth if you wanted.

- If you have a gap, it may be left for some character or closed with a number of techniques from bonding and/or braces to veneering. Small gaps should likely just be left alone.

- If you have an uneven gum line that only shows when your cosmetic dentist lifts your lip, you may be paying for a procedure so you look good for his/her pictures. Why bother?

- If the middle of your teeth does not match your face (midline discrepancy), it can be treated at great expense or left alone. You wouldn't believe how unimportant this feature really is, but how much fuss some dental professionals make over it.

- If a tooth is twisted a little, it can be treated with braces, re-shaping, bonding, or veneering - or like a small gap left for character. I'd just recommend leaving minor problems alone and instead making a donation to SmileTrain.org which treats cleft lips and palates for kids in developing nations.

This list of things you could change gets longer with the more you know about cosmetic dentistry, and the greater the range of skills of your cosmetic dentist. From doing nothing to trying to make you perfect can cost you thousands, and actually harm healthy teeth. So you really need to know if the problem is actually in your mouth, or between your dentist's ears.

TRUE/FALSE:
Being fat, or overweight, if you prefer, can put you at greater risk of significant dental problems.

Answer: Visit www.AcidMouth.com to discover the truth.

Sometimes it's NOT Your Teeth that look so Bad…it could be Your GUMS!

To me, and excuse me if I'm talking about your mama… an extremely 'gummy' smile can be very ugly. While your teeth may be straight and white if you're "all gums" like the Great White Shark in the movie JAWS, you will stand out in a crowd, and may even make people get out of the water just as quickly.

Not that it really matters what others think, but if you are self-conscious about it, you may need to have the bones of your face rearranged to relate the bones and teeth better to where your lips are. The procedure is routine for an oral surgeon, but not for the patient - so you need to be sure that it's a significant problem. Sometimes people have short lips or the lips are "hyper mobile" - meaning they move away from your teeth more than average. All this needs to be considered before you resort to surgery.

If you are very lucky, your 'gummy' smile may be because you have too much gum grown over your teeth. This can be reshaped with a laser… or, if the bone levels need adjusting too, then it is a little more involved. There is a procedure called the "Laser Gumline Rejuvenation™", of course found at the dot com of the same name which can really make a huge difference in how a smile looks.

As mentioned elsewhere in the book, some big names have done OK with their 'gummy' smiles, so you may be fine. If you are concerned about having a 'gummy' smile, dentists analyze the relative position of your teeth, lips and amount of gum that shows. We use pictures of your biggest smile (like the one you had when you heard your favorite rich aunt just died), and another picture saying "Duh" (like your high school grad picture), and also consider the length of your teeth too. You can get a quick review on RateYourSmile.com if you wish or discuss it with your dentist.

Piercing Problems

The popularity of sticking sharp needles into the lips and tongue and adding jewelry is gaining popularity. According to a dentist journal sitting on my coffee table, 51% of the people in the western world have some type of piercing, and 3-20% of the holes are in or around the mouth. My daughter is one of those statistics.

There are places on the lips that reduce the risk of damage to the gum line. A reputable piercing artist (if there is such a thing), or your dentist, will be able to instruct you where you can add ornamentation with the least risk to your health. Complications include rubbing the gums off your teeth (recession), tooth fractures, infection, swelling and bleeding.

Whatever makes your parents irritated may also cause serious risks to your health. So, if you insist on getting a tongue piercing, you should be sure to have the silicone safety balls added instead of the big metal ones. This way, when you grow out of this phase, you may still have a few teeth left to call your own.

'Veneer Nazis' can be Vicious!

This group of dentists is fussy with a capital "F". They pick each other apart in much more detail than the Real Housewives of Atlanta. They split hairs and waste their breath about things that they feel passionate about, but for the most part many of their concerns are likely things you shouldn't care less about (this applies to the Real Housewives too).

One example is some cosmetic dentists like to put little brown stains into the grooves of the white composite fillings for the molars (way in the back of your mouth). The problem is patients don't like it, because it makes the teeth look like they have cavities, or food, caught in them.

Some of the Cosmetic Academies have a "boy scout" type ranking system, and in my opinion that doesn't mean a thing. Being judged on your work by a team of cosmetic fanatics must be the ultimate humiliation. While they will disagree with my loose acceptance of natural beauty, if you want to save money you won't be fooled by anyone trying to pass themselves off as a master of cosmetic dentistry - since they may be as difficult to please as your last mother-in-law.

It's Really about the Money

Unscrupulous cosmetic dentists try to sell as many full-mouth porcelain veneer cases as they possibly can, and they rate each other by the numbers. The docs that have 'dollar signs in their eyes' can be very smooth operators and extremely likeable. Under their personable veneer, they can be predators preying on the uneducated and impressionable dental consumer.

While this group of dentists gives "cosmetic dentistry" a bad name, the public is mostly left in the dark because the profession keeps it quiet. Don't be fooled by the certificates on the wall. There are some extremely aggressive veneer dentists in the profession that wouldn't think twice about taking every penny of your life savings, as if your new smile were a life-saving heart transplant procedure.

On that note, before you get a smile makeover, ensure you and your family are covered by a reputable medical plan that covers costs - costs that would put you in dire straits if you got sick before you paid off your new teeth. You wouldn't want the cosmetic dentist to have to repossess your veneers…that would really hurt and would leave your teeth uglier than before you had them installed.

FACTOID: Who is the richest retired dental professional in the world? This may go to Robyn Moore who met Mel Gibson in the late 1970s soon after filming *Mad Max* when they were both tenants at a house in Adelaide. At the time, Robyn was a dental nurse and Mel was an unknown actor working for the South Australian Theatre Company. On June 7, 1980, they were married in a Catholic church in Forestville, New South Wales. The couple have one daughter, six sons, and two grandchildren. Their seven children are Hannah (born 1980), twins Edward and Christian (born 1982), William (born 1985), Louis (born 1988), Milo (born 1990), and Thomas (born 1999). After nearly three years of separation, Robyn Gibson filed for divorce on April 13, 2009, citing irreconcilable differences. While the settlement is private, it has been estimated to be as much as $450,000,000. Like most people know, sometimes it's not what you do...it's WHO you 'do'.

Get DRUNK and Ask a Stranger

Here's a crazy idea...go to a nightclub, have a few drinks and sit down beside someone you'd consider attractive, but have never met before, and ask them a question. Explain that you want to look better and feel more attractive, but you are wondering if what you think needs to be changed is the same thing that other people notice. There's a TV show something like this where people guess the victim's age prior to a makeover.

Assure the stranger that you want their honest opinion, and for the price of a drink you want them to look at you from head to toe and tell them the main things that stand out in a negative way. This may take a few attempts, and it may give you some surprising answers. Maybe your 'butt' is too big; you have big ears or whatever, <u>but many times you'll find your smile may not be a factor</u>.

Don't be Fooled by the Lifetime Guarantee

While I never tried to suggest my dental work would last forever, some cosmetic dentists try to increase sales by promoting the concept of a "lifetime warranty". This helps justify a huge price premium, sometimes twice the going rate. Unfortunately, as TRUMP's lawyer says of the fine print: "what the big print giveth, the fine print taketh away", and you may be left high and dry with warranty problems when the cosmetic dentist retires early - with the 'big' money you paid him!

There is enough mark up at regular fees that you should be able to negotiate a good discount and get a documented set of terms. Don't ever get any treatment over $3000 without it. If nothing else, it will help you understand what situations will be covered, and what won't be. It should state that you are responsible for proper home care and regular dental visits. Your biggest advantage is always BEFORE you commit to any financial agreements, and BEFORE you book any appointments. I guarantee it!

Chapter 4
TRICKS TO SAVE BIG MONEY AT THE DENTIST

Getting the Government to Pay for your New Smile

There are ways to 'mooch' off the government for a new smile, and when I say that, it really means fellow tax payers. If you really do need a smile makeover, and that may in fact be the case, there are several ways to make it a tax deduction.

One method is to use a "Self-directed" health insurance plan, where you are allowed to control where the money is spent. In the USA this is called an HSA or Health Savings Account. It is a tax-advantaged program with no federal tax, and you have full control because it is self-administered. The annual limits can be rolled over if they are not claimed.

A dental plan is another way people save on their dental expenses. The rules and regulations sometimes reduce how easy it is to get the specific procedure, but there are ways. For example, if your teeth are worn down you could have your teeth "re-tipped" in one calendar year, and then the cosmetic dentist can predetermine veneers or (¾) crowns the next year after you've tested the 'new look' out. The dentist can take pictures of the large white fillings, and if the edges are restored with filling, some plans will cover an upgrade.

The poor guy on the street can't do this, but if you start your own home business you can set up your own dental plan and basically get whatever you want with pre-tax money. While this won't help America get out of the massive financial hole it's in, why should you have to deprive yourself because 'a bunch of idiots wanted to burn up your tax dollars in the Middle East'?

In Canada, this program is called a Private Health Services Plan, or PHSP for short. It is a legitimate way for small businesses to allow a 100% deduction of costs of operating a health benefit plan as a business expense. The reimbursements from the PHSP to your family members are not considered income, so no tax is paid. A PHSP does not have the income restrictions and thresholds for medical expenses like personal tax returns, even though they use the same allowable medical and dental expenses list defined by the Canada Revenue Agency.

The outside cost of this program needs to be less than the tax you would save to make it worth doing, so finding the one with the lowest administration fees and setup costs is important.

I've made a huge mistake by not educating my patients over the years about this. If I were a patient that spent $10-40,000 in 'after tax' dollars on a smile makeover and I found out about this later, I'd be furious because thousands of your dollars would be wasted. Cosmetic dentists, and all dentists for that matter, need to be aware of ways they can help patients use tax write-offs.

If you need to start a small business just to be able to make this work for an expensive smile makeover, it may be worth your time.

TRUE/FALSE:
A ¾ crown costs 25% less than a full crown.

Answer: While it sounds like that should be the case, actually a partial crown or "onlay" design can cost the same or even more than the full crown. It is technically more difficult and therefore not unusual to have a higher fee. The advantage of a partial crown is that it keeps more of your healthy tooth from being drilled away which is usually a better choice.

Marry a Dental Plan

If it's not too late, another way to get affordable cosmetic dentistry, without stooping to a date with the dentist, is to marry someone with a dental plan. Marrying rich is even better...who needs dental insurance when you have cash lying all over the place?

When patients mention they are getting married, I rub my hands together with excitement…sometimes they each have dental insurance and while they are together they can use the benefits of the TWO plans! It's like taking candy from a baby, because suddenly people get their treatment almost for free.

Remember that to take advantage of this double whammy, you need to get the forms filled out, and in some cases you will get covered after living common law or if you are a gay couple. If you are gay and don't qualify, why not change your name to Pat and become "the spouse"? This may not be legal, but claiming to be the wife or husband in a relationship could be an effective strategy if your accountant and lawyer agree.

At the end of a relationship, the dental plan is almost as important as custody of the children and the pets. A solid prenuptial agreement will allow you time to catch up on those last minute touch-ups needed to get you ready to be 'on the market' again. People tend to take their plan for granted, and only when they are going to lose it do they come in and beg to get caught up, often when the time is up. Due to the paperwork, lab time, or sequence of appointments needed to do a good job, cosmetic dentistry done in a rush can usually only be a compromise.

A Lesson from the Plastic Surgeons

Recently a plastic surgeon commented that many women are getting their lips plumped up. He said "They look really good when they do a little…but some girls don't know when to stop." You know the glossy inflated 'fish lipped' look made famous by that sexy brunette on Melrose Place. She FINALLY admitted she's been getting her lips done for the last 20 years!

The plastic surgeons get haunted by patients with unrealistic expectations. Those are the ones they wished they had never treated… the ones that think that just one more procedure will make them young and attractive again. If this is your problem, you should seek professional counseling.

Date for a New Smile

Many people are able to convince the people in their relationships to finance physical enhancements for mutual benefit. How many women have had breast implants thanks to the credit card of a relatively new fling? It's not a big step to ask the 'wild-eyed' fool to also 'spring' for a little smile enhancement at the same time.

Think of the benefits for him ...how will your new look make him feel? Play up the way your smile affects your ability to love yourself and really, how can you truly love someone else when you are feeling so bad about your own self-image? Using tears can make the discussion even more effective. You'll be friendlier and bubbly and just plain more fun to be around! I'd still recommend following the advice in the rest of this book, and not just signing up for the most expensive overhaul just because someone else is footing the bill.

One final word of advice, get them to pre-pay for the treatment just in case the makeover takes longer than the duration of the relationship. (Note it as a "gift" in the professionals accounting books or he could come back to you for the money.) Be sure to negotiate a pre-payment discount with the dentist, so you can show you are helping them save money.

Buy in Bulk...even with new TEETH?

If after doing an immense amount of research, you are convinced you really need a massive amount of dental work, consider using your leverage to get a better deal. Cosmetic dentists are business people at heart and understand you have other options a short drive away.

Consider getting written estimates and appointment times so you can do the math. Could you handle doing a number of appointments at once? Maybe between you and a few others you can buy the doctor by the day instead of by the procedure code. Think buffet instead of "a la carte"!

If a "good day" for a typical dentist is $5-6000 in billings (overhead eats up most of the money) and your treatment works out to more than that (and the time needed is less than 5-7 hours) you could ask for a flat rate and <u>tell the doc you'd prefer to buy him by the day and have his absolute undivided attention</u>. You need to understand that the lab fee for any crowns or veneers will likely need to be paid on top of the professional fee, but that's fine.

While this is an unconventional idea, due to the present financial conditions there will be a few docs who will consider your offer. If your care otherwise would total $10-15,000, it may take a few consultations to get the dentist to 'swallow' such a cut. You can justify this by appearing not to be desperate for a new smile, and saying unless you get a break you won't be able to get the treatment completed.

Be sure to offer to pre-pay for the treatment, and offer to forfeit some big money, like $1500, if you need to cancel with less than 24-48 hours notice.

You can apply for New Teeth if You've been Married to an Abusive Spouse

There is a special fund set up by the AACD, which is the American Academy of Cosmetic Dentistry, which is designed to help repair the smiles of women who have had their teeth punched in by ill-tempered spouses. The *"Ike Turner" dental plan* can be a 'life-changing' experience for someone messed up by domestic abuse.

The real name is the "Give Back A Smile" program. It helps "survivors of intimate partner violence" link up with dentists and lab techs - who donate their time to provide the dental repairs needed.

Some areas have a government fund to help with medical and dental costs related to violence. The legal system can help too, if you know the identity of the offender. Small claims may be a quick and easy way to get a settlement without spending much on a lawyer.

Getting photographs, x-rays, and professional reports as soon as possible to graphically show the evidence is very important. If you wait until you heal up or cover the bruises with makeup, it may affect how much you can get. Your cosmetic dentist should be asked to provide a short written summary for a small fee , with the hope that you will return for the care. If he/she wants to charge a large amount for this kind of workup, you can likely call around and get someone else to help.

In fact, it would carry more weight in court if you did have several independent appraisals of your situation - so that that 'Judge Judy' can be assured you are not inflating your damage claim. To donate to the "Give Back A Smile" charity or to make a claim, visit: www.aacd.com.

Curse of the "Cosmetic Eye"

The "Evil Eye" is a superstitious belief which has been around for thousands of years. It is thought to cause harm to the person getting looked at by a person with such powers. Bad luck, injury or even death could occur. Various cultures found a way to ward off the evil spells which included the use of special charms, assorted rituals, and for some like Madonna (a Kabbalah follower), a red string on the left wrist does the job.

The "Cosmetic Eye" (CE) is perhaps a more serious concern. After my first 100 hour continuum training program, and a few weekend courses on aesthetic dentistry, I became partially afflicted with the "Cosmetic Eye". I wanted to veneer almost everything! Cosmetic dentists get very picky about certain details which they can quickly "fix", or actually just partially cover up with porcelain veneers. Just knowing about this distorted thought process, which affects many cosmetic dentists, can help save your teeth from being over treated.

Zip Your Lip with the Hygienist

To get the most value at your appointment with your hygienist, you need to 'sit down and shut up'. Many patients treat their hygienist like a psychotherapist and pour out their hearts as the clock ticks. Hygiene treatment is usually billed by units of time, and if you are chatting about your non-dental problems, your teeth are not getting the attention they deserve. .

There are hygienists who also like to talk. While it's great to be friendly, they are short-changing you if they constantly need to pause and share their stories with you. It's pretty tough to tell a hygienist that you would prefer that they concentrate on the job at hand without hurting their feelings. If you hurt them they may hurt you!

If you are stuck with an excessively chatty hygienist who doesn't seem to give you the care you want, discreetly let your dentist know about it. Ask if you can be booked with a different one in the future, or simply don't encourage her by giving the hygienist much reason to think you are in the mood to hear their life story.

Ask about gum problems, ask about how well you are keeping your teeth clean, and ask about the latest advances in the treatment of periodontal disease. By sticking to dental topics you'll get more out of the visit, and if you really want to excite the hygienist, ask her "How are my probing measurements compared to my last visit?"

One dirty secret you need to know is that hygienists are often used as a dentist's sales team for *extreme smile makeovers* and some actually get kickbacks for signing you up for veneer work.

Dentists sometimes FORGET their Basic Training

Once dentists become "cosmetically" enhanced, some of us seem to be lobotomized and instantly forget all our dental school training. It's not that what we learn in dental school ever proves to be that useful in the long run, but getting people out of pain, dealing with serious issues first like infection, decay and gum disease, usually should come first. That's just common sense.

It's tempting for some of us to neglect to prioritize this way and instead we may put the "big ticket" items at the top of the list. Regrettably, when cosmetic dentists 'go for the kill' it makes all dental professionals look pretty stupid when it leads to serious complications. A simple cavity may cost $100 to fill, or if neglected for a few months, it can add up to $2000 or more for a root canal and crown.

If you are going to spend so much that you will not be able to afford to complete the basic essentials within a reasonable time, then you shouldn't 'bite off more than you can chew'. Don't rely on your dentist to be especially conscious of your financial budget.

The dentist has bills too. His/hers are much more in mind when the presentation is being made than yours are. Wanting you to be "comfortable" with the cost of the treatment is really an easy way of saying the office doesn't want you to claim bankruptcy before you are finished paying. I always hate when that happens.

This same pattern also seems prevalent in new dental graduates, who are amazed at how much they can make from each additional procedure. As a patient, you need to use your own common sense to help make your dental health decisions. Start with a healthy foundation and then you can build on that.

Myth Busters Flossing Tip

Jamie and Adam on television's Myth Busters did a segment to see if dental floss could be used to cut through metal bars. Charles Manson could have been out a long time ago because apparently it is possible to use floss and a little toothpaste to saw through a prison bar enclosure. Oddly enough I recently shook hands with an actor who narrowly missed being one of the Manson victims simply by declining a party invitation from his hair stylist…now that's a 'close shave'!

If floss can cut through metal, then what I'm getting at is you probably didn't know flossing the wrong way can actually cut into your teeth. I've seen it a number of times and often the damage is quite severe. Rather than doing it the right way with an up and down movement, the sawing action if performed often enough can ruin your teeth.

While it may be a humbling experience, you should occasionally ask your dentist or hygienist to hold the mirror for you and check your flossing technique, because if you are doing it incorrectly, you may not find out until you cut into the nerve of an otherwise healthy tooth.

Bitter Medicine

If you think cosmetic dentists are going to change their *modus operandi* just because there are new advances that make many of their primary treatment recommendations obsolete, you are mistaken. Just like after the American civil war most white Southerners kept believing in their warped ideas about slavery, many 'Veneer Nazis' will stick with the party line until the bitter end. After years of dedicated training, often spending many weekends away from home and investing sometimes over $100,000 to learn a specific skill, this awakening just isn't going to happen 'without a lot of kicking and screaming'.

Many cosmetic dentists have been conditioned to have little hesitation about removing healthy enamel from their patient's teeth. And anyone telling them that this is wrong is going to get a black eye. About 15 years ago I still remember hearing a cosmetic lecturer claim that "Porcelain is superior to enamel"…justifying the rampant use of veneers. Incidentally this same cosmetic dentist is still featured on the cover of many dental trade magazines.

Internal memos warning dentists about dangers in the over-use of veneers occasionally get sent around. They are almost never 'leaked out' to the public (oops). The self-regulation and internal policing doesn't seem to make a dent, and there are still some 'crazy bastards' in every level of the cosmetic dental profession.

There may not a single "right way" to correct every aesthetic smile shortcoming. However, there are ways that cost less, are reasonably fast, and are kinder to a person's teeth than those commonly recommended by what I consider the more aggressive cosmetic dentists.

What Percentage of Cosmetic Dentists are Dangerous?

Given the choice of a general dentist or one that claims to be a "cosmetic dentist", I'd initially consider going to the general dentist if I was going to blindly follow his/her advice. Perhaps after reading this book in its entirety, you could be 'well armed' enough to make more educated decisions, and be able to see through the 'smoke and mirrors' - which are sometimes used in the cosmetic sales process.

What I consider dangerous is a cosmetic dentist who does any of the following:

- He/she follows an outdated philosophy which thinks veneers cure everything.

- Downplays alternatives to veneers.

- Uses an electronic device to somehow justify the need to change your bite with a mouth full of crowns and veneers.

- Thinks your teeth need to be as white as a preacher's collar.

- Fusses over little details and imperfections, which miraculously could be treated with porcelain veneers.

- Pressures you to spend more than you can afford.

- Makes you feel self-conscious about your smile when you really had few concerns about how it looked.

- Avoids showing you pictures of the teeth which he/she has prepared for veneers. What is there to hide?

- You only see 'before and after' pictures on the walls of porcelain veneer treatment...and very few pictures of bonding or orthodontic care.

I'd be afraid to have treatment at just any dental office, but that's the same for most dentists. *We each think we know what's best for everyone.* What percentage of cosmetic dentists do treatment that now has a better alternative than they are presently using? Don't ask me...I'm in enough trouble already. With a little additional knowledge you can gently steer a cosmetic dentist in the right direction - so he/she can save you money and still get you a great looking smile.

Specialties

There are recognized specialties in the dental profession which take a specific area of expertise and turn it into a 2-3 year program. Sometimes this makes a big deal out of something small, and one may question why dental schools couldn't routinely train dentists in a "double specialty" in the same time period to reduce the running around that wastes patient's time and money.

To confuse you even more, there are dentists who say they "specialize" in a certain thing, like cosmetic dentistry <u>which is not a recognized specialty</u>. For example, if a dentist advertises that he "specializes in TMJ"; he means he has a special focus and perhaps extra experience treating patients with jaw joint problems. Some of the most commonly recognized dental specialties you may encounter include:

- Endodontist – treats problems with root canal therapy.

- Prosthodontist – this specialist loves doing crowns and bridges.

- Periodontist – treats gum problems and often places dental implants.

- Oral surgeon – places implants, pulls teeth and repositions the bones of the face

- Orthodontist – uses braces and generally does not like to get his/her fingers wet or have to give needles.

- Pedodontist – takes care of screaming kids who have a ton of cavities

- Dental Anesthesiologist – they'll 'knock you out' and get it all over with.

If a general dentist wants you to have treatment that he can't provide, sometimes this means you'll be running from office to office. Each specialist is charging a premium, so by the time you get done not only are you spending more money, you'll be wasting a lot more time in the process. Often a general dentist, generalist or Primary Care Dentist trains to provide many of the services offered by a number of specialists, and cuts through some of the 'red tape'.

A Primary Care Dentist is like a general contractor building your new home or like a good handyman. When the job is outside his/her circle of expertise then a specialist (like a plumber, electrician, or carpenter) can be outsourced. It is the job of the primary dentist to help coordinate the treatment with other dental providers.

If you can find a specialist with a double specialty, they will be able to save you some trouble if you need the services that they offer. This saves the patient time, and he/she may offer a better rate for the "combo".

Will the specialist tell you if they think your cosmetic dentist is doing something that they disagree with? Probably not. If they do that, they are 'biting the hand that feeds them'. Dentists can get very 'snarky' with each other but it usually puts the patient in the middle and confuses matters, so most of the infighting is out of view.

Chapter 5
SECRETS YOUR DENTIST DOESN'T WANT YOU TO KNOW

Behind the White Curtain - the Wall of Silence

Dentists love to gossip and pick each other to death, but just not in public. In our minds, we see all the faults of our fellow professionals and blame the failures on the other doctor as much as the neglect of the patient. However if our own work fails, it's always the patient's fault!

Americans like to sue for everything, so dentists are trained to avoid getting people upset at their former dentist. We choose our words very carefully, and will tell you this or that is "failing" or not ideal, instead of saying what we are really thinking. What we are thinking is not always correct anyway. Keeping our colleagues out of court, even if we don't like them, is one of our unwritten rules.

Unlike lawyers who get paid to ramble, second guess and exaggerate, we are trained to do the opposite. Dragging out issues and making a big deal out of something is just a 'pain in the ass'. We'd rather have you forgive and forget and just cough up your own money to fix the problem. In the final analysis, unless the issue is catastrophic for all the hassle, this isn't always such a bad idea.

More Insider details about Smile Whitening

Smile whitening is a popular and effective cosmetic dental procedure. It's so easy that almost everyone is offering to help you. The most powerful whitening products are available legally only from dentists, or at least they should be. The dentists are fighting the unregulated kiosks that are popping up everywhere. If the concentrations of the whitening gels are really powerful enough to work in a short time, they should not be used outside a dental office.

The products can be so strong that they risk burning your gums, so applying them by yourself or at a kiosk may be dangerous. The secret behind whitening with lights or lasers is that the additional whitening from the light comes from the drying effect on the teeth. Dry teeth are whiter, so within a few days or weeks the teeth hydrate again, and you simply have the whitening that was a result of the peroxide gel.

The weird thing is that people still want the light used when they know the effect is only temporary. Even dental staff who should know better will want the light on…it's something that looks cool… and helps justify the higher cost. The actual increase in whitening power is from the stronger gel that is used during an "in-office" whitening treatment.

The stronger the gel, the better it will whiten your smile…but the downside is sensitivity. Sensitivity increases the longer the gel is on your teeth and the higher the concentration of whitener in the gel.

Home whitening gel used in trays is less concentrated, so you can probably guess that sensitivity will be lower. Will it work as well as power whitening? Actually if you do it properly and can keep it up for 2-3 weeks you will have a result comparable to the power whitening. Even though I was a cosmetic dentist, and had super-white teeth, it was because I compulsively used the home whitening gel, and in fact, I've actually never power whitened my teeth.

For many years our office was actually in the top 10% of tooth whitening sales! One of our secrets was that we kept the prices affordable right from the beginning so the average person could afford it. Low prices were sometimes thought to "cheapen" the profession and reduce the "exclusivity"…at least that was a comment by more than one cosmetic dental snob who hoped to charge high fees for everything. Like any commodity, the price has gone down with competition, so you shouldn't have to be gouged for a whitening procedure. You could likely get it thrown in for free if you pre-pay for another cosmetic procedure and 'sweet talk' the dentist a little.

If you really want to get the best results, do BOTH home whitening and the power treatment…it will cost you a little more, but if whiter teeth are important to you, it's much better to try this first before going straight for the veneering option .

Your dentist will let you know if you can expect good results. There are no guarantees, and in the end you may have to have porcelain veneers to get the color you hope for. Just remember that whitening/veneering can be addictive, and some brain-damaged Aryan Nation patients and dentists think they can never be too white. There is a point where whitening too much results in an unattractive artificial appearance. How white is too white? One expert has suggested that you check the whites of your eyes…if your teeth are whiter than that you may have gone a little far.

NEW SECRET about preventing whitening sensitivity:

By using specific gels and pastes inside your whitening trays (rather than just brushing with them) you can drastically reduce the sensitivity that comes with whitening. You can try Sensodyne® toothpaste, Prevident®, or another called MI Paste® . MI Paste is not good for people who are truly allergic to milk (not just lactose intolerant). Ideally you would use the paste in the whitening trays a few weeks before starting whitening, but if your teeth are not very sensitive you can use it after whitening or every other night.. If you just want to brush with the paste instead, remember NOT to rinse afterwards - just spit out the excess for better protection.

If You Think I'm in Hot Water by Sharing this with you - You're Right!

This book exposes what I feel are some of the biggest problems in dentistry today. Both "good" and "bad" cosmetic dentists are not pleased with any revelations about their profession. To add to this, I also will soon take a jab at the orthodontists. It's simply bad for business to have a 'rogue insider' raise 'red flags' about the procedures that 'put the caviar on the crackers'.

I do feel a little regret that some great dentists will be negatively affected by a more informed and therefore suspicious public. The wariness may lead patients to request less ideal dental care than they should. That's definitely not my intention…I just want the public to know they need to learn more about the new breakthroughs that are making traditional cosmetic dental procedures obsolete in many situations, and secondly, you can't always trust a cosmetic dentist or a dental professional just because he/she is a lecturer or a world renowned cosmetic trainer, or because they have a fancy advertisement.

My venture into exposing embarrassing occurrences within the profession has resulted in repeated and multiple threats to my staff, slanderous comments to my patients, negative comments online and on the radio, attempts to cut off my access to dental supplies critical to providing care to my patients, voluminous complaints from competitors to the dental association, online blackballing, and hundreds of thousands of dollars in legal threats. When I was selected "Best Dentist in the City" I was accused of cheating by an anonymous competitor and reported to the association. To top it all off, I even got a large Mexican burrito mashed into the side window of my luxury SUV!

All the 'crap' I've been subjected to has made me 'one mean hombre'… irritated enough to shares things you'd usually only read in secret code if you had a dental degree.

The Pictures Your Cosmetic Dentist would be crazy to show you!

While we could have done a full color book and loaded it with scary pictures you'd likely miss the point. Instead we have posted the graphic gore photographs on the book's official website at www.ConfessionsOfAFormerCosmeticDentist.com and all you need to do is type in the CODE (CFCD) to see graphic pictures of the damage a 'Veneer Nazi' can inflict on someone's healthy teeth. While teeth usually need to be prepared for veneers, when they start out perfectly healthy I protest loudly (unless I'm holding the drill, then I just look over my shoulder a little more often). While the photographs are actual samples taken from dental magazines, they are almost NEVER shown to the public, because they would obviously have a huge negative impact on sales. Once you see them it will make you think twice before having an aggressive *extreme smile makeover*.

Be sure to sign up for the FREE e-reports that can get you 'the scoop' on developments that can help save your smile, and literally thousands of dollars. We will also give you much more information that we were unable to include in this book due to space limitations.

Bad Cosmetic Dentists

While few would admit it publicly, many dentists in the aesthetic branch of dentistry, loosely called "cosmetic dentistry", are concerned about the ones who seem to have lost their common sense. 'Veneer Nazi' was a term I thought would get attention and express my opinion of them at the same time. While I'm one of the few who would go on the public record and admit it, many talk openly at dental seminars and in dentist online forums about the problem.

The two biggest concerns expressed are:

1. the damage to healthy teeth and
2. the gouging of patients' pocketbooks by doing more treatment than they really should. Those themes are repeated many times within this book (but some people are slow learners), complete with specific examples and warning signs.

The difference between a "Good" cosmetic dentist and a "Bad" one is a matter of opinion. I've seen some cosmetic dentists get standing ovations from huge crowds of dental professionals. After seeing what they were doing, I thought they should get the gas chamber (100% nitrous oxide- death with a smile). The dental profession has 'pockets of madness'. Who should you believe?

I would suggest it is safer to be a little skeptical of everything you see, read or hear. America is great at selling almost everything, and something that may be good in one situation may be a crime in another. Any time you feel pressured into a smile makeover, it's a warning sign. The cost may not even be a factor for you, but simply because you can drop $40,000 onto a new smile doesn't mean it's the right thing to do. The rich can be as stupid as anyone, and being arrogant because you can afford something… can get your teeth in trouble.

Just like too much plastic surgery, too much cosmetic dentistry as a psychological way of pampering yourself can be a mistake. A good cosmetic dentist should be ready to talk you out of treatment that he/she feels is wrong for you. I didn't always invest enough effort in this, and sometimes it would come back to haunt me.

STOP- Print off the SPECIAL REPORT: The 20 Reasons Why A Cosmetic Dentist Should NOT Just Do Veneers! (Visit our website for details)

This detailed report will help your dentist understand there are many new things to consider before jumping into a traditional smile makeover. By giving your cosmetic dentist this report from the "Confessions" website, it will make them aware that you are not simply an uninformed potential 'smile makeover victim'. You can even go over the report point by point to see how it relates to your situation. If the cosmetic dentist dismisses the report as a bunch of "crap", I strongly encourage you to change dentists immediately and seek a second opinion from a respected practitioner in another office. This information is not something I just made up out of thin air, it has been distilled from some of the most respected authorities on dentistry, and can help protect you from doing the wrong thing.

An Online Rating Lawsuit & Plane Crash Claim Combo

A few years ago best-selling dating book author Ellen Fein was sued by a NYC cosmetic dentist for $5 million dollars. She called him a quack and alleged that he ruined her teeth. Posting the notices on LyingDentist.com and BadDentist.com got her into some hot water.

I contacted the author to see what the latest update was, and was informed she couldn't really say anything about it, but the suit appeared to be dropped or settled. A few years later, the same dentist sued the estate of New York Yankee baseball player Cory Lidle for $7,000,000, after the plane the pitcher was piloting crashed into the apartment building where the cosmetic dentist lived.

"Can't You Just Veneer My Teeth?"

While this used to be music to my ears and meant I'd be able to cover another month's lease payment on the Lamborghini, now it means

<u>I failed to get my patient to understand that veneers are rarely the first thing to consider for cosmetic dental treatment.</u> I'm not saying these people are stupid, but sometimes I just don't have time to give them enough information to change the mental block that they have. Sometimes I call in another dentist for a second opinion, other times I hit them with 'the gore book'. If it's close to lunch time, I just tell them I don't do many veneers anymore, so if that's what they want I pass them on to another more cosmetic-type dentist. The pre-conceived notion in the brains of most of the general public or laypeople as you common folks are called, is that porcelain veneers are the 'be-all and end-all' in cosmetic dental care…this in my most current opinion is simply dead wrong.

Porcelain veneers are simply chips of porcelain which are stained and glazed to look something like enamel. They are not enamel and they do not form a perfect replacement for healthy enamel. They are not as harmless and reversible as getting a set of artificial acrylic fingernails. Once you finish reading this book you will have a different outlook on a smile makeover. Hopefully you will be able to avoid unnecessary treatment, and be able to see through 'the hype' that has permeated the mainstream media.

What would 'Suze' Orman say?

I'm not sure if Suze has ever gotten this question from a caller, but let's try imagining what she'd recommend for this caller if she had read this book:

Caller: "Hi Suze…I just visited my cosmetic dentist and he said I need to get about $47,000 worth of dental work. I don't have the money but I am thinking about re-mortgaging the house to do it…what do you think?"

Suze: "OK, so your smile sucks?"

Caller: "I didn't think it was bad until the dentist showed me what I looked like on his computer"

Suze: "Are you in a relationship or not?"

Caller: "I'm married and have two kids…my husband never complained about my smile before."

Suze: "I don't care who this cosmetic dentist is, if you are married and you are pulling money out of your house just to have a new smile you're probably the dumbest caller I've had today. Get your dental care up to date but don't be talked into spending money that is in the equity of your home. Grab a brain!"

Suze usually lays it on the line and I'm going to be brutally frank with you - regardless if I offend you or your dentist. Coincidently, just as I'm typing this, Suze took an actual call from a woman (More Best Calls You've Never Heard), who was asked to co-sign to cover for a sister's loan to cover her dental work. She recommended that she just say "no" because she wasn't in a position to easily afford it. Good advice Suze!

The Top 7 Ways to tell if a Cosmetic Dentist is a 'Veneer Nazi'

If you can avoid making the mistake of following the wrong cosmetic dentist's advice, you can potentially save $22,000-$47,000 or more.

Take the test that follows and see what you discover (answer Y/N beside each statement below as you read):-

1. Your dentist suggests that your teeth are not white enough, even though you think they are fine.

2. You have a small space between your teeth and the dentist thinks you should close it with veneers.

3. Your teeth are healthy and a little crowded, so your dentist suggests veneers.

4. You have one crown or veneer that doesn't match your teeth so your dentist suggests doing all your teeth.

5. You have a discolored front tooth after root canal treatment and your dentist suggests doing veneers on all your teeth.

6. You want a wider smile (like Julia Roberts), so your dentist suggests building out your teeth with veneers.

7. You have occasional headaches, so your dentist suggests using a machine to give you a new bite and a mouth full of beautiful veneers.

If you've answered "Yes" to any of the questions above you may want to look at other alternatives before doing a 'bank roll' of veneers. Alternatives may include simple combination of a number of treatments including whitening, bonding and orthodontic braces/aligners, or doing nothing at all. There is also another type of treatment that may also be particularly effective which we will discuss in more detail later.

If you feel an uncomfortable feeling of financial pressure during a cosmetic dental examination, it is usually best to give us a simple 'out' by telling the dentist your own version of following:

"You've given me a lot to think about in terms of treatment, cost, warranty issues, complication risks and long term risks...I'm going to think about it and discuss it with you again. I especially enjoyed the step by step pictures of the process involved. For the time being, can we start with some basics...like a cleaning and getting that one cavity filled before it gets worse?"

Alternatively you can claim to have a bad case of 'projectile' diarrhoea and a nail appointment across town for which you're already late. This will usually clear the cosmetic dentist out of your way quite rapidly!

Try to refocus the cosmetic dentist on the essentials, and avoid getting pressured into something you are not really sure of. I often made the mistake of only offering the patient the most expensive alternative, and this is a technique that was taught at a particular cosmetic training program which I'm not very fond of now. The most expensive option is often the WORST option for the patient, and simply easy money for the cosmetic dentist.

Insider Dental Report Exposed

In a recent letter to dentists, a major cosmetic training facility stated many myths were circulating about their style of training, and they wanted to 'set the record straight'...these are some of the concerns they feared were ruining their reputation:

1. Their dentists didn't care about their patients.
2. Their cosmetic dentists only do cosmetic dentistry and place veneers.

3. The cosmetic dental practice can't survive since it doesn't accept insurance.
4. Their dentists over-diagnose.
5. They only do full mouth veneers.
6. They only care about money and they charge excessive fees.
7. They drill down the teeth too much.
8. These dentists only treat the rich, and avoid the poor.
9. They make the teeth look too long.
10. The group is a cult.
11. They use a machine to help them decide how much dentistry to do.
12. They try to teach how to do a full mouth of veneers after a weekend course.

Years ago, I attended a number of courses offered by this company and I was not impressed by them at all. I think they are better now, but if cosmetic dentists attended the earlier programs and haven't updated their beliefs, I would be fearful for their patients. I was even an understudy with one of their gurus, who was fixated on the idea of using the "myo-monitor" (an electric pulsing muscle relaxing device), which is used as their 'magic' machine to justify a new bite position. My former instructor used to advocate using orthodontic braces to achieve the magic bite while the cosmetic program recommended using veneers. Coincidently, the course was sponsored by one of the biggest porcelain veneer labs in the world …hmmm, I wonder if there is any connection.

Jaw Joints: Nobody has ALL the Answers

While one group uses a magic TENS machine to pulse the muscles (into a position they call Myo-Centric), another group who is their sworn enemy uses a pushed back jaw position (called Centric Relation or just CR) as a starting point. One of the leading experts on this alternative position admits that most ways will work most of the time because people adapt. Heck, you can even cut a person's arms and legs off and some will keep on rolling along. Nothing ever works all the time, and even the "pushed back" jaw position is not exactly a stable spot, and people often function slightly outside any special/secret/proprietary area that any group of dentists prefers to claim as correct. .

Dentists need to have something to believe in and a starting point to help them build a person's teeth. The fact is, most changes need to be tested to see if they are going to work out. My bias, as you can easily see, is against any style of care that pushes people towards a very expensive treatment alternative or is used as an excuse to do porcelain veneers.

If you do have "TMJ" problems we may post a link on the book's website to a practitioner who could help you or include it in the free e-reports.

Why You Should OVER-PAY Your Cosmetic Dentist

There is a huge secret that I'll share with you that will blow your cosmetic dentist over…*offer to over-pay him!* Why would this be a good idea? The answer is quite simple, in many cases it is easier for the cosmetic dentist to make a whole load of porcelain veneers match (basically ear to ear veneers), than it is to fix a single tooth in the middle of your smile with one veneer.

It is often said that doing a single upper middle tooth (a central incisor) is one of the cosmetic dentist's biggest challenges. So the dentist may unconsciously be afraid of the difficulty, and try to convince you to do your whole mouth. If you know your other teeth are in pretty good shape, before the doctor goes too far in the long winded sales presentation, try this line:

"Doc, I know you may think I need a new smile…but I've been doing OK with the one I've got. The fact is, I probably get laid more than you do! Sure, I wouldn't mind doing a little whitening first, but how about if we just veneer the ONE tooth to match all the others? I know it will be a bitch to get the color just right, but I'm sure you'll be able to get pretty darn close. In fact, if you can do it in less than two or three tries, and it blends in with the others, I'll be willing to pay you a 50% premium."

This will certainly have the dentist speechless for a few moments.

Resist the urge to say anything (the silence will add to the drama)... he'll catch his breath and realize you know much more than the average 'makeover' patient. Your homework will 'scare the crap out of him', and he may even suspect you have a hidden camera and are doing a story for 20/20. That's good...in fact he may even decide you are too challenging and call off the whole thing!

So by offering a 50% premium, or say $1500 for one veneer (over the average $1000 fee), you could save $6500.00 if he was trying to sell you on eight veneers... and you'd save $8500.00 or more if he had his 'big boy pants on' and was trying to close you on a 10-unit porcelain smile makeover.

By offering to pay more, you can save BIG...something you can put in the bank and use to put your spoiled kids through college. Aren't you glad you bought this book?

Beware of the Commissioned Staff

You are on your own in the office of a cosmetic dentist. While the staff may appear warm and caring, many times they are motivated by a financial incentive tied to what you decide to do to your teeth. If you could see inside the staff room, you would possibly see a list of their names and a daily total of the number of porcelain veneers they "sold" each day.

Knowing this can help you stay on guard and it will remind you to take their "independent advice" with a grain of salt. They are not trying to mislead you. Thanks to brainwashing courses, they truly feel you need a better smile, but they have additional motivation to ensure you forget about your other financial obligations - like food and shelter.

Dental staff can get all kinds of perks including trips, cash bonuses, gifts, uniforms, sick pay and medical coverage. They often even get free porcelain veneers so they can be used as smile models. After a while the staff starts to get lazy and needs to be re-focused on the business side of the cosmetic dental office. There is no better way than a commission or bonus tied exactly to what the cosmetic dentist wants to sell you...**veneers!**

Chapter 6
THE PARADOX OF CONSERVATIVE COSMETIC DENTISTRY

The Cosmetic Dentist versus an Average General/Family Dentist

I would feel safer seeing a "good" family dentist than one that heavily promotes him/herself as a cosmetic dental expert. The risk of seeing a cosmetic dentist who is too aggressively biased towards the use of veneers would make me averse to the idea of venturing inside one of their offices, and simply accepting their treatment unquestioned.

Many superb cosmetic dentists admit within their ranks there are too many dentists that are veneer crazy. I would rather have slightly crooked teeth than have any type of veneer treatment, including the "no drilling" style of veneers that are increasingly popular.

A dentist who simply is listed as a general or family dentist is less likely to be focused on selling veneers. While the dentist may still provide a veneer makeover, it will not be pushed on you in the same way as you would experience by the manipulative, over-zealous and scripted sales techniques of some "high end" cosmetic dentists.

If in doubt it is better to get the basics healthy, and postpone any major cosmetic overhaul…or at least wait until the cosmetic dentists learn more about the recent breakthroughs that make veneers a last resort. I have talked to a number of dentists who have the same concerns that I do about this issue. Many of them try to correct the damage patients receive after an aggressive 'smile makeover', but there is no way to go back. I hope you bought this book in time.

Conservative Cosmetic Dentistry and Other Lies I told My Patients

I used to think I was being conservative and telling patients the truth when I said they needed veneers, but this was only because relative to crowns, veneers WERE more conservative. Rather than drilling away all the enamel from the teeth (like I would do with a crown or cap preparation), I only drilled away most of the enamel from the front, sides and tip of the tooth. I thought it was "conservative" because I left most of the enamel on the inside of the teeth.

Hopefully I left some of the enamel on the front of the teeth because the veneer tends to stick to it better, but in reality I would often drill away more than I should have. Once we start drilling, it is difficult to stop, because a dentist always likes to dabble with things to make it better. The lab tech needs to have room to build the veneers so I learned to drill away more than I wanted to.

I would explain that I only needed to reshape the tooth a little for the veneer work and the thickness of a dime was all I wanted. Much of the time, it ended up being closer to the thickness of a nickel, and as far as teeth go, that can be 50-90% of the thickness of the enamel.

I tried to avoid letting the patient see the prepared or "drilled down" teeth...actually I bent over backwards to try not to let the patient see the stubs! "Stubs" was one of the words we banned in the room while the patient was there, but sometimes it slipped out. If a patient felt the teeth with their tongue, they would often say, "Wow there isn't much left". My pale-faced reply would be "it feels worse than it is," knowing in reality it didn't look very pretty until the temporary veneers or the final veneers were cemented on.

If patients wanted to go to the bathroom in the middle of the procedure I had them slip on a pair of Depends® adult diapers (instead of letting them check out their drilled teeth in the bathroom mirror). It was like walking on thin ice.

I also briefly discussed the need to wear a night guard after having veneers, and didn't go into great detail about all the precautions until AFTER I had bonded on the porcelain - fearing that maybe it would affect the sale. 'Bagging' a set of veneers was a pretty big deal, and compared to doing fillings, it was fast money.

I now regret many of the veneers I placed, and will burn in cosmetic dentistry hell for an eternity; unfortunately, I'll have a lot of company.

Makeovers Sell like Cocaine and are even Addictive for a Dentist

A 'smile makeover' is a seductive offer that often exploits a patient at a point of weakness. The person sometimes feels ugly, lonely, or is grasping for something to help them attract attention. Recently divorced people are a common target for a makeover...this trade secret may get me killed before this even goes to print. The glamour and sales skills I used as a cosmetic dentist could be almost irresistible, and many times patients would be ready to cash in their life savings to get a new smile.

I found that most patients could easily be lured into thinking their teeth are not white enough or perfect enough. This is in spite of the general looks of the dentist giving the cosmetic advice - who may be fat, bald, short, wrinkled, pale or 'geek-ugly' (I have a little of each). Cosmetic dentists can use special verbal skills to make even the most glamorous feel inadequate...and that's the optimum time to "go for the jugular".

I confess that I still have occasional "cosmetic dentist" relapses, and have the urge to drill down people's teeth, but for the most part I am able to control it now. There are no support groups for former cosmetic dentists, but writing a confessional book is about as close as it gets.

Quality, Service & Price

Everyone wants top quality dental care, amazing service and low prices... but is this possible? According to most business experts you simply can't have it all without having to pay for it. It is possible to have short bursts of any combination of the above, but in general the more you pay, the better the quality and service should be expected to be.

Dentists tend to think they are better than they really are, with 90% feeling they are in the top 10% regarding quality rankings. Luckily for dentists, patients are almost totally in the dark when it comes to judging quality, so if we get along with someone and they think it looks and feels OK, then we've gotten away with whatever we did.

According to a recent study from UCLA, 18% of patients choose their dentist based on the technology, so if the dentist has a 'gizmo' that impresses them, they think the dentist is a good choice. It's not always that smart an idea because often the 'gizmo' is not that great an innovation, and if it is amazing the dental professional may not know how to use it very well.

According to the same UCLA study, more than six per cent of new patients pick their dentist based on ethnicity and language capabilities. Certainly, it is important to have the dentist know what you want done, but there is little relationship between the languages spoken and the quality of care. It may be better to bring your own translator and see the best dentist you can find, than to find the ethnic dentist who is not known for their quality or best bedside manner.

Price is the number one reason males choose a dentist, and over 33% of new patients overall choose their dentist based on price. Other factors include distance to the dental office (12%), dentist recognition (10%), extra services (6%), and being a specialist (6%). The internet is becoming a significant source of new patients, while the Yellow Pages are used less and less.

When it comes down to it, some people are fooled into thinking that the more they spend, the better the result will be. They even get snooty and say dumb things like "MY dentist charges $ ____ for this or that" as if it was somehow better. It may be better or it may be worse...a patient would rarely be in a position to know any better.

Promises of MASSIVE Wealth

Cosmetic dentistry was something of a dentist drug during the last 20 years. A dentist could become like a plastic surgeon, creating beauty and changing people's lives. There were also promises of huge profits...in fact, some lecturers bragged about charging one patient as much as what many dentists would charge hundreds of patients over a whole month.

Justification for such 'bank robbing' fees was made, and we were brainwashed into thinking we deserved big money. Cosmetic dentists were often trained to sell the big case, 'go for the kill', and offer very few, if any, alternatives. Why waste time with little people with little problems when you could "specialize" in cosmetic dentistry and just do veneers all day at $1000.00 to $2000.00 per tooth?

A story we were told was about the artist Picasso. It went something like this…a person asked Picasso to do a sketch for him. He obliged and within a few minutes he had it done, then he asked $10,000.00 for it. The client asked, "How could you charge that much for something that took you less than ten minutes?" Picasso replied, "It took me a lifetime to be able to do it." Our specialized training, while sometimes learned over a weekend, put us psychologically on a pedestal.

One lecturer justified our potentially massive fees because we were just as important as a sports star…why shouldn't cosmetic dentists make as much per hour as a guy who dribbles a basketball? On paper, every cosmetic dentist theoretically could drill down a tooth every 10 minutes for a veneer if every patient and mammal within reasonable driving distance of their practice "needed" 32 veneers. Perhaps then the average cosmetic dentist would be able to live in the same neighborhood as Michael Jordan. But the main reasons for getting us pumped up into Veneer Gods was to sell us on taking more cosmetic dentistry courses, and to hire the sponsoring dental lab to provide our patients' veneer lab work.

While few of us weekend "cosmetic dentists" became super-rich, the courses began to distort our thinking and we began to look to our labs as the true cosmetic experts and that put our patients at risk. The labs and the companies running the course made the real money, and should have been more responsible. On the other hand, the dental professionals who attended the courses should not have allowed themselves to be 'sucked into' this scam.

The Holes I've Missed

Like Charlie Sheen…I regret the holes I've missed filling over the years. Being what I thought was a cosmetic dentist, my focus was what could I do for my patients to make them look better. I started to look at decay and gum disease as a nuisance and sometimes didn't look hard enough.

Tooth decay can occur in very obvious places, and sometimes in the weirdest areas that are almost impossible to find. The light doesn't get there, the tongue or cheek is in the way, the patient is drooling or gagging or belching…you sometimes need to make it quick and make a best guess. Often x-rays are not put far enough back, or forward, or they are taken at the wrong angle, so the information is sometimes less than ideal. Rather than ask for another x-ray, I would sometimes hope for the best, but this sometimes meant a cavity got missed. It was embarrassing to see a patient a few months later with a toothache from one of these oversights.

Other times, gum disease would sneak up on a patient with pretty good habits and the occasional tooth would be pulled. Once in a while the extracted tooth showed how much tartar was missed by the hygienist. It can be very tough to get the hardened minerals off the roots, especially when the gum disease progresses. Sometimes the hygienist would probe down thinking they were at the bottom of the gum pocket when actually they were sitting on a lump of tartar (calculus)…so it was a tough sell when we told patients they needed a deeper cleaning after they just paid for one. The fact is, over the years I missed a lot of problems and suspect most dentists occasionally make the same mistake.

Oma's Cosmetic Dentistry Horror Story

My mother-in-law, who we call Oma, is over 91 years old as I write this. She's one of those sweet old ladies that everyone 'loves to pieces'. In her day she baked and cooked the most amazing German delicacies you could imagine. She survived World War II in Germany and worked herself to the bone, maybe even saved a few Jews.

How she fits into a book about cosmetic dentistry is that she used to have slightly crooked teeth. Over half a century ago, things were a little different, and her dentist recommended that she get an upper denture to give her a prettier smile. Her teeth were healthy, but they were just a little crowded, so what the dentist did by pulling 14 good teeth was essentially a crime.

She has now lived half her life without her real/natural upper teeth, and her blind faith in her dentist's recommendations is something she continues to regret to this day. Oma would probably kill him if he wasn't already long since mummified. A denture may be the answer for someone with an extremely messy situation, but hopefully it is no longer used as a quick fix for a cosmetic problem that could be corrected with more conservative techniques.

There is no "set age" that people need to get dentures, and you should expect to have your own teeth even as the mortician pumps formaldehyde into your veins and Crazy Glues your lips together. In the same light, porcelain veneers have been used improperly on thousands of patients in the last 20 years, when we really should have known better.

Don't Fall for the Testimonials

Let me tell it to you straight…reading a bunch of fancy testimonials that say the cosmetic dentist is fantastic is not a reason for you to accept the recommendations. We are becoming very sophisticated in the use of testimonials, which help build confidence in the services we promote. By law, testimonials can even be revised a little as long as the change does not modify the essence of the message.

Be skeptical of any cosmetic procedure, and remember, many of the testimonials have been coached to "tell an emotional story" that will suck you in. If you watch any infomercial you'll see the same process, they show you a great product, you hear a number of testimonials, and then you have all kinds of incentives to buy.

Just hold off a little longer before you get that 'smile makeover' there is more you need to know.

The Right to REFUSE Care

You need to know that you have every right to refuse or post-pone care that you do not want, can't afford or do not understand. It is difficult to tell a dentist you don't want to do something, but the doc would prefer you to be honest than to go along with a recommendation then complain about it later.

Ask a 'ton' of questions, and if you are not satisfied, get a second opinion.

Chapter 7
EMBARRASSING PERSONAL EXPERIENCES & MORE INSIDER SECRETS

Lotto Winner

When one of my patients won six million dollars in a lottery, I was a little jealous. I had recommended quite a bit of dental work in the past, and I thought she'd be ready to jump on board and get it all done and then go on her world cruise. After her win, I thought I deserved to charge her more, maybe $10,000 per tooth. I guess its human nature to want to steal from the rich and keep some of their "easy money." I guess that's how lawyers start to think.

To my amazement the savvy lotto winner asked me to pre-determine the treatment to her dental plan to see if it would be covered. I think I may have sniveled something under my breath, like "Oh God" or something like that. I felt it was ridiculous that she wouldn't just pull out a huge roll of bills and pay for what I told her she needed.

Many rich people let their teeth fall apart. One of my cousins from Iowa just bought a tractor and a combine for the north side of $500,000 US and when he smiles he is missing every other tooth on the right side of his face. He's so cheap that he even used to drive an hour up to the dental school - to get the more affordable dental work, instead of paying full price at his regular dentist.

When you win the lotto, it's probably best not to brag about it at your next dental appointment, just get done what you think you need - because if a crazy cosmetic dentist smells money, you may be getting more than you need.

XXX Sex Talk at the Dentist

Maybe I'm a little old-fashioned but I won't be having the following discussion with any of my patients:

"STDs are transmitted during unprotected oral sex through open wounds, non-intact oral mucosa, blood and saliva. In fact, millions of teens become infected each year through engaging in unprotected oral sex. Sexually transmitted diseases such as Chlamydia, gonorrhea, HIV and herpes infect young people each year because they believe oral sex is safe." (ref: Abuse - by C. Yellen)

The report mentioned above recommends that dentists should consider addressing "risky behavior" with patients who show signs of oral lesions that may correlate with sexually transmitted disease. It's a little late by then, don't you think?

Rather than having this awkward discussion with the dentist, you may soon see a sign on the ceiling above each dental chair. The placards would simply say, *"If you give BJ's or are thinking about it, please discuss it with the dentist first."*

The Revealing Mirror on the Wall

I was always trying to add a little 'touch of class' to our dental office without spending too much, and one time I saw this really nice mirror with a deeply carved golden frame that I just had to have. It was a little large, but we hung it on the wall anyway.

The mirror faced the patient when they sat in the dental chair but there was one big problem…when we dropped the patient back the mirror gave us a view of the patient's underwear (if they were wearing a skirt or a kilt). Fortunately, we treated very few Scotsmen at the time, but I knew I couldn't keep the mirror due to this issue. As much as I liked the mirror, there was no way to find a place for it that didn't put patients at risk of a potentially distracting "Brittany Spears-limo" fiasco.

Interview with a Victim of Cosmetic Dentistry

In my many years as a cosmetic dentist, one of the worst stories I heard first hand was from a dental assistant who wished to remain anonymous - out of fear that talking about it openly would affect her future employment. She had been enticed to be "the patient" for a dentist taking a cosmetic dental course, sponsored by a popular program.

She explained the dentist had to fly her to the course in the city (I won't say where exactly because they'd probably sue me). The cosmetic training project was to prepare her front teeth for porcelain veneers. In most veneering treatments a portion of the tooth is drilled away to allow for the thickness of the material. Generally, most of the healthy enamel is stripped away from the front, edge and sides of the tooth being treated.

The poor tooth takes quite a beating with this procedure and her teeth were drilled down, then the instructor was called over and they were drilled some more. Then the dentist touched them up a little with some more drilling and finally molds or impressions were taken for the lab work required.

A day or so later the lab work came back, and the veneers were tried in and cemented on. Something went wrong and whether it was the fit or the color, it was decided that they needed to be remade.

This was not good as the second time they were re-made, not only were the veneers drilled off, but even more of the remaining tooth structure was ground off. This always happens each time dentists need to do things over again, and we don't give it much thought.

The dental assistant happened to peek in the mirror to see the stubs left over by the dentist's drill…she was horrified. She was left with next to nothing of her original teeth. She began to cry and even years later she still tears up and turns red in the face, re-living the experience.

Her teeth have never been the same. While they look fine from the outside, they hurt, and some of them may even need root canal treatment.. She says "I wish I had NEVER done the veneers in the first place!"

FACTOID: Patients who have moderate to severe wear on their teeth can often be easily and affordably treated with a special composite filling material that is stronger than most brands. Think of it as "retreading your tires" rather than buying exotic new ones. In the author's opinion, a dentist can use composite rather than temporary acrylic crowns or veneers and still have excellent results. The brand of composite and before/after photos/videos are revealed on the website.

The Problems with Some of the MOST COMMON Choices in Treatment

One of the greatest advances in dentistry has been the development of dental bonding. With the ability to actually stick porcelain or composite filling material to a tooth, the dentist is able to control the shape and color.. The drawback is that most veneering procedures involve a certain amount of enamel loss, as the tooth is drilled away to make room for the thickness of the veneering material.

Why should you worry about losing some enamel? It is there for a reason…to provide a hard protective coating that grinds up food and protects the nerve from harm. By drilling away the enamel the tooth is weakened, and the ceramic material which replaces the enamel does reinforce the tooth, but it is not a perfect substitute.

The problems with ceramic materials used to veneer teeth include the following:

1. Porcelain cracks easier than enamel. The human body is an amazing thing; and evolution has provided us with the hardest coating produced by our own cells for the outside layer of our teeth. Millions of years ago some lucky organism stopped eating things whole. It formed some lumpy hard things in the orifice that was to become its mouth which, when rubbed together against food, made it easier to digest. In respect for nature's years and years of trial and error, it's usually best to keep as much of your own enamel as you can.

2. The joint where porcelain or bonding meets your tooth can stain. This can make your veneers look ugly and a warranty may not apply.

3. The joint area between the porcelain and the tooth can leak

and decay.

4. The porcelain can wear the teeth or dental work that it rubs against. While most of the modern porcelains are smoother than they used to be, there are still problems with having different materials chew against each other.

5. Porcelain chips a lot easier and is not easy to repair. So, if a person has a grinding habit, they may be in for additional replacements over the years. Tooth grinding is very destructive, and while we do discuss it in greater detail later in the book, you need to know any tooth that is ceramic is at extreme risk of breaking if you are a heavy tooth grinder.

6. As you age like your hairline, your gums will recede, and the edge of the porcelain may not look very nice. While the cosmetic dentist may make the edge of the veneer just at the edge of your gum line, or even a little ways under your gums, there is no way to anticipate or compensate for the amount of recession or "shrinkage" your gums may have in the future.

7. Porcelain does not whiten, so if you whiten your teeth after having veneers you may get some mismatched colors. Sometimes we forget to ask patients if they want whiter teeth until we've already prepared the teeth for veneers. The best time to whiten is months or at least weeks prior to the veneer process.

8. Once you do a few veneers, you usually end up doing more later on to make all your teeth match.

9. It is very difficult to match the color of teeth with an artificial material, and under different lighting conditions the ceramic materials may be quite obvious.

10. Veneers cost a fortune. At almost $1000 per tooth, the average veneer wouldn't be too bad if it wasn't for the fact that some cosmetic dentists try to 'upsell' you to at least eight to ten of them.

The advantages of porcelain over composite veneering materials are primarily stain resistance and a "slicker" surface. The cost of porcelain is usually quite high, and sometimes the veneered teeth take on a fake look, especially in photographs where flash bulbs are used for additional lighting.

I do not want people to think for one second that veneers are not an amazing cosmetic procedure which can totally transform a hideous smile. There are certainly some excellent situations where veneering procedures are appropriate. The most common application would be when a patient's teeth are already heavily filled from previous damage, or the condition of the enamel is poor. A new surface can work wonders just like a fresh coat of paint on a wall.

The problem with veneers is not the procedure; the main problem is they are sometimes overused when other procedures are more suitable, or they are used as a shortcut with results that are less than ideal.

Why would a cosmetic dentist suggest something that is not appropriate?

Here are several reasons:

(i) It's the procedure they feel they are more competent at performing. Cosmetic dentists have traditionally been taught creative but fairly aggressive ways to avoid orthodontics/braces.

(ii) The dentist has been hyped up with the amazing power of a specific veneer by a course, and is excited about trying it.

(iii) The dentist does not know the twenty reasons why veneers should not be done until other factors have been considered. .

(iv) The cosmetic dentist does not know or pretends not to know about the latest advances that make veneers less appropriate.

(v) The dentist may make more money doing one procedure, and not make any if they send you elsewhere for something he/she can't provide.

(vi) They are overly concerned about the concept of perfection, and diagnose treatment which is totally focused on taking your smile to an imaginary point which does not respect the idea of natural variation.

(vii) The cosmetic dentist is attempting to pass a cosmetic organization's board exam and has to show he/she is a perfectionist.

"Be who you are and say what you feel. Because those who mind don't matter. And those who matter…don't mind" - Dr. Seuss

Snap on Smiles?

There is a product that is a fast and cheap makeover for people on an extreme budget. Given the choice between jumping into a porcelain makeover and having to sell your body on the street corner to pay for it, or choosing an affordable 'quick fix' of clip-on teeth, it may not be such a bad idea - even though there are options which are much, much better in the long run.

Simply put, these snap-on appliances fit over your teeth, and are easily removable when the party is over. They give you a new smile, and although it's nothing like the real thing it is a way to test a new look to see if it's right for you.

It's difficult to say what type of person should consider this without being insulting. To be nice, I'd only recommend it for a short term solution for someone who is very short on money, and needs to have a better looking smile… maybe for a job interview or that first date with the hot and interesting person you've been chatting with online. In the USA with its growing lower class and shrinking family budgets, this option may become pretty popular. Visit SnapOnSmile.com for further information.

Magnifying Glasses

I was one of those dentists too cheap to buy the "loupes and lights" that brain surgeons use. I also was worried they would ruin my eyes and blind me. Once I finally got a pair, I never went back to squinting; it was like seeing for the first time.

Even with the big overhead lamp, dentists still have a difficult time seeing. The 'funny looking' magnifying glasses really help, and in fact there are now dentists using microscopes allowing dentists to work upright (so hunch backed old dentists may soon be a thing of the past). The cost is coming down, and they are more for an office who just sees a few patients per day, but there are probably specialists who would not want to work without them.

While some cosmetic dentists would disagree, I wouldn't say a dentist is bad because he/she doesn't use this high tech magnifying technology. They just may be a little behind the times. We are experimenting with an idea called "Dentistry in the Dark" where the treatment room is dimmed, and most of the light used is focused inside the patient's orifice (mouth). It is more relaxing to have the darkened room, and in fact it is almost romantic...the only thing breaking the mood is the rubber gloves, masks and glistening stainless steel (but some people are into that).

The darker room helps the dental team see better because the light outside the mouth is distracting. If your dentist has a great view overlooking the city or the ocean, that's great for him but not for you. The distractions are one thing, but looking at your x-rays and seeing the problems in your mouth are actually much more difficult in a bright room. Once your dentist goes dark, she won't go light again.

TRUE/FALSE:
Dentists use lasers to detect tooth decay.

Answer: There is a laser cavity finder that has been proven to be better that a dentist's pokey pick (called an 'explorer').

Dental Employees from Hell

Running a number of dental offices for a few decades has made me jaded. I've been able to stay relatively relaxed in spite of having to employ liars, thieves, gossips, whiners, embezzlers, procrastinators, insubordinates, flirts (well, that was a perk), and people who dragged their personal problems into the office. There is even a website for reporting the worst offenders at www.DentalEmployeesFromHell.com.

Dentists can be weird, staff can be insane, and patients can be psycho too. In some cases like attracts like, and everything works out fine. Other times one of the participants is not like the others and the mix can be a disaster. The neat thing is that the crazy people think the normal ones have the problem. You know the feeling when someone cuts you off while you're driving, and then flips you the finger...or even pulls out a gun and 'blows offs a few' in your general direction. It's kind of like that...you can scratch your head and think about it all day, but it's better to 'get the hell out of their way' even when you are right.

I've got my share of "bad" staff stories…like the assistant on her last day of work who I caught packing her pockets full of floss. Or the assistant that forged one of our dentist's signatures on a prescription for narcotics…perhaps she had a bad migraine, and didn't want to trouble him with the risks of getting writer's cramp. Oh, and the assistant that stole from another assistant's purse and then asked her to give her a ride home. We've seen all kinds.

Getting a background check before hiring someone seems like a very good thing to do these days, especially when you are dealing with money and people's health. Con artists and incompetent people are everywhere, and your dentist may or may not be doing a good enough job to keep these special folks out of your mouth and your wallet. Ask your dentist if they do background checks on their employees, and I'd suspect much like myself until only recently, they would lie and say "of course".

If you Love your Teeth… then Don't have Kids

Women know having babies takes its toll on their bodies, but their teeth can suffer almost as much as their rear ends. Gaining weight, vomiting and heart burn seem to welcome the newly expecting mother. Vomiting shoots stomach acid up into the mouth and the low pH dissolves the enamel right off the teeth. Enamel doesn't reform, and each time a person throws up they lose a small amount of the protective coating sometimes with very serious complications.

The acidity increases sensitivity of the teeth, but more importantly it can lead to thin enamel, changes in the bite and the look of the teeth, and it even increases the decay rate. Cavities can quickly grow into the nerves, and result in the need to have a filling, root canal or extraction.

The old wives tale of "lose a tooth for every child" is often a reality if women avoid routine dental care and do not take special precautions. If you are pregnant, the best time to visit the dentist for routine care is during the second trimester, or anytime before the contractions begin or the water breaks if you are having problems. A veneer makeover is rarely a good idea during pregnancy. Visit AcidMouth.com for more information about the damage related to stomach acid.

How Technology Helps To Sell Dentistry

Intra-Oral Cameras…a GREAT Way to Sell You More Dental Work

I knew I could scare the heck out of a patient if I could just get a good picture of their teeth. If a tooth is cracked or has a big ugly filling, but it's sitting in the back of someone's mouth, it can be tough to convince someone to spend money on repairing it. People have no idea what is going on inside their mouths.

It's for that reason that I usually had my dental assistant take a close-up photo, and maybe add a few "gasps" followed by something like, "Oh my GOD!…Your tooth has a condemned sign on it!"

My favorite technique is a full close up 'smile picture' taken by the assistant and put on the big computer monitor. I'm not in the room, and actually prefer to wait and give the patient time to really get a good look at what they look like close up. Naturally, I have a picture of a perfect smile on the wall to show them how they could look…all they need to do is ask.

Before & After Computer Tricks

I almost bought a program that showed patients how they would look if they signed up for veneers. It was in my days of being a cosmetic dentist, but I was worried the final result would be not quite as perfect as the pictures suggested.

Computer imaging allows a dentist to "photo shop" a new smile to get a patient excited, sometimes about the wrong choice of treatment. An excited patient often wants something NOW and does not want to listen to all the pros and cons… <u>they want to look great before the weekend!</u>

Before and after pictures can be helpful, but be careful to ask about the procedures that are required, and see if the dentist explains about as many alternatives as possible, especially the more conservative ones .

FACTOID: Cosmetic dentists look at ways to use veneers to make teeth "look" straighter, while orthodontists look at ways to use braces to actually move the teeth into a better position. It is difficult for professionals to move from one perspective to another.

Over-Kill with X-Rays?

The latest thing in x-rays is getting 3-D radiographs and CAT scans of a patient's head. Some experts feel these types of x-ray machines can be over-used when simpler ones will be sufficient . The exposure to radiation is much higher with these exotic devices, so they should be used only in certain situations: for example, if a patient needs a number of dental implants, and the dentist/surgeon is wondering where they should be placed within the complex structures of your head.

If you are just going to a dental professional for routine care you likely do not need to be exposed to this procedure. If you do get one of these expensive images taken, you should ask if the fee includes an evaluation of all the details by a certified radiologist who has specialized training in this exciting technology.

High Tech Digital X-Rays are WORSE?

Recently a dental guru confirmed what I suspected for years…the fancy digital X-ray programs dentists are now buying actually are not as accurate as the old fashioned ones. The advantage of digital x-rays is a 7-9 times reduction in the amount of radiation used, but the ability to actually see tooth decay is poor when compared to the old style film x-rays. *In fact, dentists may only see half the initial cavities that you actually have*!

So if you don't regularly go to the dentist, some of these holes could sneak up on your nerve and give you a surprise in the middle of the night. So sometimes high-tech advances don't always make improvements in every feature, and that should open your eyes to the need to take some personal responsibility. Brushing, flossing, fluoride, and regular dental visits still apply as much now as in the old days.

White fillings grow Man-Boobs?

There has been a big scare in the news in the last few years about a chemical in white dental fillings called Bisphenol A. It's used in the production of plastic bottles, epoxy resins and it's used in the food and beverage business. It has been suggested that the chemical mimics a female hormone, and it can lead to breast development in men, and links to heart disease and diabetes. In the final analysis, there may end up being a problem with everything a dentist wants to stick in your mouth, but a few white fillings and sealants probably won't take you past an A cup, or make as much a difference to your health as the artificial butter on your theatre popcorn.

The REAL Problem with White Fillings!

Aside from a little controversy about the chemicals that go into the fillings, what I find to be the biggest concern is that most of the white fillings that have been put into people's teeth over the last 20 years are starting to break down, and many times they were used inappropriately.

A few years ago when TV shows were freaking people out about mercury silver fillings, dentists and patients rushed to the next cheapest alternative -composite or what some people simply call "white fillings". Remember the dentist on 60 MINUTES that scared the public about the risks of using mercury silver fillings? His studies found that sheep got higher mercury levels in the brain if they had more fillings. It did raise concerns about the silver amalgam that we were all trained to use for simple fillings and many patients began to panic.

When we started using more white fillings in the back teeth, I began to see some problems. I can still remember actually seeing the teeth crack before my eyes, as we hardened the fillings with our little lights. The white fillings used 10-20 years ago actually shrunk so much they damaged the teeth. Now many of those white fillings are falling apart or have been replaced already by the next generation of white composite filling material.

Composites should really be used for quite small restorations, but most dentists use them almost any time a patient does not want to upgrade to porcelain or gold restorations. Porcelain fillings/restorations are made outside the mouth, usually by an outside lab, and bonded into place on a second appointment. The porcelain does not shrink but it can chip. Generally, the bigger the restorations are, the better it is to have them made outside your mouth "indirectly" - but new advances can change this rule of thumb very quickly and white fillings are becoming more durable and often can compete with the more expensive alternatives.

Flaws in Modern Ceramics

Porcelain has been used in cosmetic dentistry for a long time, and technology keeps coming up with improvements. Sometimes the improvements are sold to dentists before the bugs are worked out. That may mean for you as a dental patient that some of these new crowns may break sooner than we expect.

The problem with the popular white zirconia crowns (zirconia is a super-hard white material) is that a weaker porcelain is baked on top of the inner core. This smooth layer sometimes flakes off and results in a broken crown/cap. These types of crowns are a 'bugger' to drill off because the inside core is so hard. The old standard porcelain fused to metal crowns can still be pretty reliable, but they may not look quite as nice.

A recent dental article reminded me that there is actually a good reason to use metal-free restorations like zirconia (or the new e.max CAD crowns which may have a lower failure rate than the zirconia brand)… especially for women. Women commonly have allergies to the metals used in dental work, and this can result in redness of the gums around crowns with the offending metals. According to an expert in the field, 50% of women are allergic to copper, palladium, nickel, chrome, or gold, which are the same metals used in dental work and jewelry.

Gold is still a favorite material of mine, and likely the best wearing and most durable dental material, but it is mostly used in inconspicuous areas in the back of the mouth. So even when gold prices are sky high, gold crowns may be the best value for your money because they are so durable - and if they fall out you can actually cash them in!

Dental Terms & one that they BANNED us from using…

The tooth language, jargon or terminology dentists use is naturally confusing to someone who doesn't understand it. I still don't know half the big words academic dentists use (like gums are called gingival, but I keep forgetting if gingivae is plural or singular). Let's review a few of the most common terms to help you understand what dental professionals are saying behind your back:

Molar relationship:- it's not whether your back teeth love each other or not, it's just a little bite assessment to help tell the doc how your teeth fit together.

Overbite:- just the overlap of your upper teeth down over your lowers…if you have too much overbite you are dying (just kidding, well I suppose we are all dying, hopefully very slowly). Many people mistakenly confuse it with the next word on the list.

Over Jet:- another measurement of your front teeth, how far your top teeth stick out ahead of your lower teeth.

Incisors:- your front biting teeth (four on the top and bottom)

Canines or cuspids:- these are the fangs that vampires use to suck blood, and cats use to clamp down on mice so they can't escape.

Bicuspids:- these are not teeth that swing both ways unless you have serious gum disease, they are usually the next two teeth past the canines counting back into the darkness of your mouth.

Molars:- molars are the big grinding teeth at the back of your mouth which generally come in about every 6 years after birth until you get a third set. So at age 6 you get your first permanent molar behind your baby molars; age 12 you get your second molars behind the first set; then add 6 to 12 and exactly on your 18th birthday just after you finish your last tequila shooter… "splurt" …your four wisdom teeth come in.

Baby teeth:- primary teeth or milk teeth are the first set you got.

Extraction:- pulling or removing a tooth

Gingiva:- the fancy term for your gums (but you know that already).

Gingivitis:- inflammation or infection of the gums

Periodontitis:- gum disease that has spread deeper into the gums/bone around the teeth

Probing:- measuring the little gum space around your teeth

Decay/Cavities:- rotten, stinky holes in your teeth

Attrition:- the amount of wear on your teeth (usually caused by grinding or acid issues)

Root Damage/abrasion/abfraction:- damage to the root of the tooth near the gum line

Shade/color:- the dental team can check the color of your teeth, and if you are an A1 or B1 you are OK, if you are an A4 you will never marry.

TMJ:- your jaw joint (some people have TMJ problems)

Bitewings:- little side x-rays taken to check for decay.

PA:- "Pee-ayes" are little x-rays that show the root of your tooth if they jam them in far enough

Panorex:- an x-ray that buzzes around your head and gives a panoramic view of your teeth, sinuses, and some of the bones in the area

Ceph:- an x-ray of the side of your face to check your profile

Study Models:- plaster models of your teeth used as paper weights and to study how your teeth fit together

Wax up:- a simulated change made in wax on a model of your teeth that the dentist may propose to you to make you look better, and have a chance at finding a mate.

Mesial/Distal/Buccal/Occlusal:- all kinds of words that tell the dental people what part of the tooth they are talking about…sounds better than front, top, inside, back and let's us charge more for the time we lost in dental school.

The word that was banned from this book would have gone here… it was a word so secret and so volatile that it would have given the author more notoriety than the writer Salman Rushdie – who, after writing Satanic Verses, had to go into hiding from Muslim assassins. The benefit was the 'weird-looking dude' ended up with some pretty hot chicks after the book came out.

After careful thought and several threats from the orthodontic and cosmetic dental community we have decided to avoid the use of the term within this whole publication. Please do not write in and ask for the word as once you know it, "it" will have the potential to take over your mind and potentially ruin your life. It is a word that becomes obsessive, and you would never look in the mirror again in quite the same way. You would lose something precious that you would never be able to regain. This is hard to explain but trust me this is a word better left untold.

We can only hope that our restraint in not using the dental word "_____" in this book was a wise decision. Sometimes the less you know, the better. If pressed under interrogation, there is no doubt given enough time and full use of electricity, blunt and sharp trauma, water and chemical torture, sleep deprivation, starvation, solitary confinement and country music, the word could theoretically be extracted.

If you are a trained dental professional then you know the word (although you may not know it unless I tell you, but once I told you it would be "Oh ya…I know that word") and you would know why I am not using it. Something we can share is the secret dentist password for the word…it's "Oprah gets lost in the Caribbean". Maybe I better change the subject, I hear ADA helicopters in the distance.

Chapter 8
CELEBRITIES & THEIR FREAKY SMILES

Cosmetic Dentists can Change your Life and make you a Success?

Behind every successful person there is a cosmetic dentist…that's why they are always thanked at awards ceremonies. There is a feeling of power within the cosmetic dental community which can only be partly justified. We can help people who are affected by lack of confidence in their smiles. Dentists can make an ugly smile more attractive. This is truly a gift of cosmetic dentists that is as rewarding emotionally as it is financially. Unfortunately cosmetic dentists who don't know when to stop can also take a nice, natural looking smile, and make it look artificial with too much treatment.

There is also a problem with the kind of thinking patterns that many aesthetic dentists seem to develop. Cosmetic dentists sometimes put too much emphasis on the minute details of an "ideal" smile, as related to a person's ability to be successful or be attractive to the sex of their choice. If you want to have a nicer looking smile, that's great…but unless you have a distractingly ugly smile, a new smile probably won't make as much a change as you hope it will.

Celebrity Smiles … a closer look

Before we gently part their lips and pry into the mouths of some of the best known celebrities of television, sports and the National Enquirer, let's talk in more general terms about them behind their backs. Most of these high profile people featured are not much different than you and I...they just have more people looking at them - both the celebrity and the parasites clinging to them make a living from our intense infatuation. The parasites may have fancy names and degrees like agent, lawyer, accountant, marketing rep, makeup artist, body double, security guard, publicist, manager, personal consultant, financial advisor, PR department, personal shopper, personal trainer, housekeeper, yard keeper, pool attendant, private jet pilot and crew, and of course, all the relatives and friends that suddenly become very needy after the celeb hits it big. They are like a prize winning show dog with loads of bloodsucking ticks...as quickly as they chew one off, a few others hatch.

These famous people are always under the microscope. They are under scrutiny about everything they do and say...and of course, what they look like and smell like creates trends among their followers. Some people stop bathing because some guy in a movie they like did that, and sadly, some are inspired to do hideous acts like driving a hybrid car after watching a Gore movie.

What the public doesn't know is the dental profession joins in on this microscopic inquisition, and naturally zooms in on the teeth. Here's a taste of what typical dental professionals would say about some big names and a few stories about celebs and dentists.

Michael Phelps and why he could never win at the Olympics

Michael Phelps is the US swimmer that seems to always be in the news, he's the guy who proved all the dentists wrong...a mouth breathing guy with a weird bite could win 14 career gold medals at the Olympics and hold numerous world records. If orthodontists had it their way, he would have had thumb-sucking appliances, speech therapists, braces and probably oral surgery, before he even had his pool pass.

Of course, there are many ways people can get this 'career stopping bite condition' besides mouth breathing, big tonsils and thumb sucking. If Michael has his mouth around a 'bong' as much as the media makes it seem, then this could be the problem.

Phelps could not have earned $1,000,000 from the Speedo Company if an orthodontist was on the board of directors. Luckily for him, that was not the case.

Tyra Banks the 'snaggle-toothed' Super-Model

If you have a dental degree, and a certificate from a non-recognized specialty from a cosmetic dental association, you will be able to look past Tyra's stunning good looks and focus on a huge flaw…her crooked lower teeth. Only Andy Rooney from 60 MINUTES has more unsightly lower incisors than she does. He's the old guy on the news magazine program who makes small talk at the end of the show. Andy and Tyra probably have the same dentist.

How could Tyra go so far, and get so rich and famous, with lower teeth that are jumbled up like a car pileup on the interstate? Her teeth are so crooked 'they make Clay Aiken look straight'.

Just because Tyra was the first African American woman to be featured on the cover of GQ, the Sports Illustrated swimsuit edition, and was voted Super Model of the Year, doesn't mean her teeth were perfect. Another model with crooked teeth is Isabella Rossallini…she was canned from her Lancôme fragrance job not because of her twisted teeth, but due to her age. Obviously dentists are not part of the screening process in Hollywood (or are never consulted by advertising agencies).

The Tom Cruise Smile

Here's a guy that's gone from the TOP of the charts to the Bottom of the popularity polls, and back up again. His smile has been on more magazines than almost any movie star, but the cosmetic dentists and orthodontists shudder and use him as an example of a "midline" gone wrong.

The middle of Tom's smile is off to one side a little bit…or put another way, the vertical line between his top front middle teeth is off to his left - in relationship to the middle of his face. If memory serves correct, he had a tooth taken out on one side (one of his bicuspids), and the remaining teeth shifted over. Orthodontists and cosmetic dentists have talked about Tom's midline even more than the fuss about him jumping on Oprah's couch!

Of course his flawed smile blew any chances that he'd ever be selected for a magazine cover as Sexiest Man of the Year, or that he would be the 'lead' in movies directed by Steven Spielberg. Dentists almost become paralyzed at the sight of his grin, and use his smile all the time as an example of how important the midline of a smile is.

Hmm....maybe it should be how <u>unimportant</u> the midline really is. In the real world we are not put into symmetrical graphic analyzers and discriminated over a few millimeters. We are judged when discrepancies are larger...like when your right ear grows out of the back of your head, or that kind of thing. You can use these unique features to withdraw from society, or you can celebrate your oddities and make millions starring in block buster movies.

The Late Michael Jackson Was Ripped Off at the Dentist?

Recently a dentist from Ireland told me a story about how the late MJ almost got swindled by one of his kid's dentists. According to the 'doc', MJ's childcare helper took one of his children in, and the dentist said the youngster needed about $37,000 worth of dental work. Fortunately for MJ, he was a little suspicious and had someone else take his kid in a second time, in disguise and under a different name. This time the child only needed $700 in dental treatment.

The biggest dentist 'rip off' against Jackson was by the late Dr. Evan Chandler who alleged his son was molested. Now that the former Beverly Hills dentist committed suicide, the victim supposedly has come forward to say it was a setup. At $20 million, it was likely one of the biggest individual dentist scams ever and the story behind it will make a very interesting book someday. Oddly enough I recently met an orthodontist from Hollywood who knew this dentist and was shocked to hear of his death.

Dentists are only human and some fall prey to their dark side and modify their prices and advice based on their perception of the patient's net worth. We are taught from childhood in Robin Hood stories that it is OK to steal from the rich.

The simple fact is rich people actually want to pay more for things because they think they are getting something better. Why would a dentist want to argue with that? In fact, if you want to learn more about this concept check out the book "Marketing to the Affluent" by Dan Kennedy. It's a great read whether you are a patient interested in being an entrepreneur (so you can actually afford a smile makeover), or a cosmetic dentist who wants to cater to the rich and famous.

Crooked like Beckham

David Beckham is that English soccer star whose name is synonymous with the sport. While I may have watched parts of a game or two on the "telly", it was at a Spice Girls concert in Los Angeles where I first saw the 'soccer god' in the flesh. He was a few rows back at the foot of the stage extension, keeping a smiling watch on his slim wife Victoria, as the girls rocked the Staples Center. A newly pregnant Nicole Ritchie was up in the stands, and my cousin Matt and I soaked in the experience. The concierge at the Modrian Hotel on the Sunset Strip had found us some aftermarket concert tickets a few days before, and the seats were awesome.

Anyway, that Beckham is one good looking 'dude'. The rest of us guys may as well go home, or at least stay off the field. However he has one weak point…something that should have stopped him from ever getting a 'bazillion dollar' contract and 'gazillions' in endorsements, and even his own cologne. His teeth are crooked by anyone's standards, but the cosmetic dentists and orthodontists are gasping for air and clutching their chests…for them, it is a cosmetic dental 911 emergency.

Here's a guy who has twisted teeth and yet his face is featured in close up advertisements for some of the most prestigious products in the world. So maybe his boyish good looks overpower his English teeth… or maybe a certain amount of crowding is perfectly acceptable - until you move to LA for too long. Unless he gets this book in time, he'll eventually fall victim to an *extreme smile makeover* and he'll never be the same again. Do us mere mortals a favor and keep just one tooth a little twisted, won't you Beck…just to show the dental smile experts that life accepts some features that are less than perfect.

David Letterman and How He REALLY Got the Gap…

While cosmetic dentists all used to think Dave got his gap from sucking his thumb, or having an abnormal swallow (called a tongue thrust), we now uncovered the truth. He was nibbling excessively on his female staffers, and like any oral habit it can have an effect on the teeth.

Dave is an original guy…his goofy smile suits him perfectly. The space between his teeth is something dentists call a midline diastema, but we'll just call it "the gap." You may notice his tongue dart out like a 'drugged rattlesnake', or like a baby who just tasted some spinach-flavored pabulum for the first time. He works it into his routine quite well.

I may have crossed paths with Letterman in NYC once…a ball cap and a little grin not quite showing his trademark gap prevented me from a positive ID…but I'm pretty sure it was him. If he fixed his teeth, nobody would recognize him.

Other Gaps

Gaps in celebrity smiles have stalled the careers of many…Madonna, and even Arnold Schwarzenegger (who had to drop out of show biz and go into politics to make ends meet). You'd think these people would have their people get a hold of a reputable cosmetic dentist or orthodontist to fix their gaps…I guess not.

Even the famous female aviation pioneer, Amelia Earhart, went missing before her cosmetic dentist could fix her gapped smile. For some reason Hilary Swank gave her character in the movie Amelia a repaired gap which should have been digitally recreated for authenticity. According to documentaries on her life, she was well aware that the little space would affect her marketability, and was coached not to 'smile too big' for the cameras. In a weird irony, the gapped-toothed pilot was featured in a GAP khaki pants advertising campaign.

Patients often come in with concerns about spaces between their teeth. The space may be small, but to some who have become fixated over the issue, corrective treatment is an option. If the teeth beside the space are a little narrow, then bonding or veneers may be the most appropriate. When the teeth are already a nice shape, and width and widening them to close the gap would make them look more like a couple of pieces of Chiclets® gum, or like the character played by Jim Carey in the movie MASK, then moving the teeth together with orthodontic braces is the best way to address a space (the one we call a "diastema").

The drawback of moving the teeth is that they generally need to be bonded together to prevent them from repelling each other later on. That is, unless you are willing to wear your retainers more than the average person. The relapse of the dreaded gap has frustrated many patients, dentists and orthodontists, and has likely contributed to the high suicide rates in the dental profession.

Kyra Sedgwick - Curse of the Reverse Smile

This actress has cosmetic dentists pouring cement over her Hollywood Star of Fame almost every day of the week. When Kyra smiles she barely shows any teeth, and actually has what cosmetic dentists call a "reverse smile". Her upper middle teeth seem to be shorter than the ones on the sides, which is the reverse of what they should be... to be "esthetically correct".

If the Academy, or should I say the American Academy of Cosmetic Dentistry, had their way, she would be stripped of all those Golden Globes and People's Choice Awards. They would have also forced her to have a smile enhancement and could have ended up as a stunt woman for Julia Roberts.

Her biggest curse was not her smile (which could be instantly revised if she really cared, by re-tipping her incisors in a one hour appointment for some composite bonding...no freezing required!) but instead, her greater worries include being ripped off by Bernie Madoff's investment scam.

Anthony Bourdain...No Reservations at the Orthodontist?

This food connoisseur from New York is featured on television critiquing exotic meals from around the globe. The most obvious concern from a dentist's perspective is he never seems to have the time to straighten his lower teeth. If he flossed, he'd probably find more hors d'oeuvres than most of us see in a lifetime. Garlic, chives, pig head, chicken feet, bone marrow...this guy has a fridge full of freaky stuff caught between his teeth - that would have made Jeffrey Dahmer's mouth water.

Despite the protests from orthodontists and cosmetic dentists across America, Anthony continues to enjoy success and fame...he is even allegedly married. Apparently some unlucky woman has to kiss that mouth of his (she must close her eyes and pinch her nose). This is just another example of someone with unsightly teeth slipping past the dental censors.

Ellen Barkin

This blond movie star is famous for many roles - including playing a sexy dame in *Sea of Love* with Al Pacino...but her smiling lips are so crooked that dentists get sore necks watching her in even a short scene.

Her sexiness is not scientifically possible...symmetry is the general rule. Every dentist and cosmetic surgeon tries to make their patient's left and right sides as mirror images of themselves. There must be a reason we have to be the same on each side but I couldn't find the textbook that explained it very well. I guess in nature the deformed beasts were less promiscuous as part of the natural selection process.

That probably explains why Cindy Crawford was dropped as a Supermodel when they found a mole on just one side of her face. Anyway, for those of you who are still attracted to Ms. Barkin and may chance on a date (according to reliable sources she is apparently newly single ...but this could change with the next tabloid issue), you may want to refrain from excess humor, which may provoke Ellen's trademark crooked smirk, which could very well ruin the whole evening.

Michelle Obama

The First Lady has a smile that at first glance to the untrained eye would appear to be just fine...filled with big white teeth. However, upon closer inspection, there may be some serious concerns. Her teeth show when she isn't even smiling...which is perhaps a good thing for a politician's wife who has to help instill confidence regardless of how bad the economy is.

This smile condition is called "maxillary excess", and every orthodontist and oral surgeon in the world understands those 'word$'. Although her smile may greet heads of state and some of the most powerful people in the world, she has a smile deformity which is detectable and measurable. Her teeth are a little crooked too...and while we are in the White House anyway, the President's gums are a little grey from his smoking habit. What's up with that? If George Bush had to give up booze and cocaine, why can't Obama give up nicotine? Dark gums could just be pigment (there is a rumor that Obama may be black), or it could mean less oxygen in his blood and poor circulation in his gum tissue…not good signs.

Another big name with big teeth that resembles Mrs. Obama is actress Alexx Woods - who plays the medical examiner on CSI Miami. Her upper teeth look like they might jump out and bite one of the corpses… but this didn't stop her from getting the job on TV. Finally, another actress who has upper teeth that hang down below her lower lip, at least in some advertisements (in this case inside her lip) is Andie MacDowell… incidentally she has a spokesperson contract with the cosmetic and hair color company – L'Oréal. (Obviously cosmetic dentists, oral surgeons and orthodontists were unavailable for comment).

Joe Biden or 'No Biting'?

The current vice president of the USA was known as the poorest politician…the reason…he spent all his money capping his teeth. Some lucky dentist retired early thanks to Joe and left a mouth full of artificial looking porcelain crowns in his wake. Only the actor Gary Busey has uglier looking dental work.

Joe may speak his mind, but he certainly has to be careful what he bites into with all those crowns. Porcelain, as we have explained, is not the perfect replacement for enamel. It looks pretty good from a distance, but it chips easier and doesn't put up with ice chewing or peanut brittle very well.

If you are thinking of crowning your teeth, don't make the mistake Joe did…choose a color that doesn't distract from your speech, one that doesn't create a reflection as bright white as Conan O'Brien's 'butt'. Pick a color that maybe would be found in nature. Real teeth have a little more translucency than Wite Out® and actually have minor imperfections. Joe's a good guy, but his dentist's lab technician really needs to change the formula for his porcelain.

John McCain and the Grind of Politics

The loss of his race to win the presidency was not due to the bumbling mistakes of his former boss, or the lack of experience of his 'hot' running mate, it was due to the yellowish color of his teeth, and the amount of wear he displayed with every forced grin.

John's jaw muscles are so large that his bite force would likely compete with that of a hyena, or maybe even Bethenny Frankel (from the Real Housewives of New York City). His big jaw muscles may have helped him escape from Vietnam. Few people know that McCain actually chewed through the bamboo bars and ate his captors alive. The stress of years of imprisonment would show itself every night in his dreams. The nightly clenching and grinding (called *bruxism* by dental professionals everywhere) has leveled his teeth, and shortened them into stumps.

His "poor" wife must be half deaf from the grinding noises every time John McCain hits the sack. Just a crazy suggestion, but he could see a dentist for a whitening treatment and a night guard appliance. While he could have done much for America and turned the country around from the 'nose dive' as easily as Obama, he couldn't compete with Barack's trademark smile.

FACTOID: The author recently met a dental professional who claimed to have made a night guard for Leonardo Di Caprio. So even big stars wear dental appliances "just like us".

Katie Couric & Gwen Stefani …Gums loaded?

They're paid millions every year, but when these gals unleash their full smiles - cosmetic dentists cringe. These gals have what dentists call a "hyper mobile lip", and that means they have more gum showing than Ed the Horse. If you made as much money as they do, maybe you'd be smiling like that too!

A study by an orthodontist has determined that a specific maximum number of millimeters of upper gum tissue has been found to be attractive. I prefer to see Katie smiling with all her gums showing rather than trying to hide her quirky grin with a conscious effort.

Ghosts, Guns and Scary Smiles

That actress who plays the woman who sees dead people and helps the police…hmmmm …there are a few to choose from…..oh, yes… Patricia Arquette, now she's got a smile that Hollywood cosmetic dentists would never accept! Yet somehow she got on a TV show about ghosts, and so did Jennifer Love Hewitt who has a 'perfect set'… and her teeth are pretty nice too. Like the Canadian rock chick, Avril Lavigne, or the Dirty Harry star, Clint Eastwood, if you have a smile like this you'll never amount to anything!

Another actor, director, musician, Emmy & Golden Globe winner who could never amount to anything with this type of smile is British comedian Ricky Gervais. He even played a role as a dentist in the movie Ghost Town…but he could have played an even bigger role as a "cosmetic dentist" if he had his teeth fixed first.

This smile is called a "Class two Division 2 smile" by dental keeners who can spot this deformity from the nose bleed section of the audience. Talk about a smile of the lower class…only the Class three smile with the big chin is worse (…that's why Jay Leno got canned, 'don't ya know').

The Clint Eastwood smile…with its upper middle teeth (central incisors) pointed back and one or both lateral incisors pointing forward, smaller lower jaw and all, that would mean you'd have to 'pack a 44 Magnum' to get anywhere in life.

Of course, orthodontists and oral surgeons can help these people with extensive treatment, and hopefully few complications (like a numb lip that doesn't even feel the dried breakfast cereal left on it throughout the day)…but stubbornly, these celebs are too busy making movies, doing concert tours, and directing Academy Award worthy films to keep their 'damn' dental appointments. The dental profession can't help those who continue to refuse treatment!

The Kennedy Curse…Bad teeth

While the family had a time in the American limelight, their smiles left dental professionals in the dark. Jackie Kennedy had a smile that would shock members of the American Dental Association. It's the same kind of smile that we discussed above. Orthodontists would have recommended lengthy correction and possibly jaw surgery…she would have been black-and-blue and wired shut for half the first presidential term.

How would she become the prize of Greek billionaire "Ari" Onassis, and yet still not have the funds to correct her crooked teeth? Imagine how loved and rich she would have become - if only her 'jagged chompers' could have been straightened sometime along her journey. Certainly an orthodontist on Martha's Vineyard or in Manhattan could have done 'the poor gal' a favor.

Maria Shriver's Kennedy genetic programming gave her lower teeth as crowded as Grand Central Station during the morning rush. She had to marry a guy (Governor Arnold) with spaces between his teeth to be able to kiss. There is no way she should have become a prime time television news celebrity with incisors like that. Invisalign® dentists wouldn't have a chance…she'd need a few extractions to even make a dent in the project.

Maybe between Arnold's spaces and Maria's crowding, their offspring will finally break the curse and be able to blend back into society with the rest of us.

That Crooked Bastard on The Sopranos

Damn! Speaking of crooked/crowded teeth, the actor that keeps getting movie and TV parts thanks to his ugly teeth is Steve Buscemi. He's perhaps the only actor that should be allowed to keep his freaky smile - so dentists have someone to point to, and make fun of. He's played Tony Soprano's cousin, Tony Blundetto, in the HBO series and all kinds of odd characters.

The way his upper canine is squeezed almost completely out of his mouth is so bad it could be used as a can opener. Orthodontists and dentists flood the actor with hate mail as he thumbs his dentition in their faces, and acts as if he can have a full fledged acting career without a Hollywood smile. "Good for You!"…anyone trying to break into Hollywood should stop trying to be perfect and go there as real as possible. Your chances of getting 'a start in the biz' are much better that way.

Richard Gere

American gigolo movie star, pretty woman 'womanizer', and husband of a couple models… the guy has somehow managed to sneak under the radar of the American Orthodontic Society. The 'on screen' close-ups make Richard's crowded teeth so huge that the sight has caused many dental professionals to walk out of theaters in protest.

You'd think if the Dalai Lama was so honest and enlightened, he'd pull Mr. Gere aside and say in a soft tone "for Buddha's sake man, get some braces on those ugly lower teeth". No. That doesn't seem to happen, he continues to get roles thinking a full head of silvery hair and sexy leading ladies will distract dentally trained audiences from the malalignment of his 'little biters'. Those superfluous things may fool the commoner, but to the dentally inclined, he will never be acceptable until he submits himself to cosmetic dental correction.

FACTOID: Television's "Ugly Betty" show has continued to discourage adults from getting orthodontic treatment, when it is often the best decision they could make. Braces come in porcelain varieties that are almost invisible, but they are generally safer to use on the upper front teeth than on the lowers. Ask your dentist/orthodontist about it or visit our website for more information.

Amy Winehouse and Tooth Rot

This English music artist has let her dental care, along with her life style, wash down into the gutter. She's an example of why you need to keep yourself and your kids off drugs. The crack dealers should start selling dental insurance to cover the horrendous damage that their chemicals inflict on the human dentition.

It's sad to think that a cosmetic dentist hasn't taken the opportunity to woo her into a 'smile makeover', in turn for more than a little press… HELLO!!! Somebody help this girl. Rehab can come later…we're talking about some serious tooth damage here.

William Hung

This buck-toothed singer set the world on fire a few years back - with his rendition of "She Bangs" on American Idol. As exciting as watching a person have an epileptic seizure in the checkout line at Wal-Mart®, this guy was special and had absolutely no pride.

Dentists and orthodontists classify him as a class 2 division one bite… which is a situation where the front teeth stick out, and the lower jaw is small. You risk losing an eye if you bump into these people. Not very many people have become big name celebrities with this look…he's the only one that comes to mind, besides maybe Bugs Bunny.

Mr. Hung was kept in the running for a short time as a gesture of goodwill thanks to Paula and Randy. These few moments of celebrity have helped the odd-ball entertainer originally from Hong Kong get a few movie rolls, release a couple of albums, and snag a handful of advertising jobs.

Our emails offering a complimentary 'smile makeover' to Mr. Hung have yet to receive a response. Of course it would be the dumbest thing he could do!

Sir Richard Branson can't afford a Dental Plan?

Entrepreneur Richard Branson may be too busy building companies and flying in the stratosphere to get his teeth checked. He smiles as if he doesn't even know he has two sets of lower teeth packed-in together like a shark, and seems to have a crowned one on top that could have been put in 'by a street dentist from Pakistan'.

No offence, but he gives the English a reputation for bad teeth. If his breath is as bad as his teeth, you'd expect he'd never have to worry about a prenup because who would marry him? If he did squeak one past the current wife, let's hope for his sake he sought the advice from an expert on BillionairePrenup.com.

Not only are his teeth mismatched, crowded, and yellow, they are also worn down quite badly. It must be stressful building all that wealth, but you'd think the successful businessman could afford a dental plan upgrade above the basics (provided for free in the UK). If you're reading this Sir Richard, Virgin Dental Plans™ is available for a starting bid of one million English pounds.

Marilyn Monroe

Almost 50 years after her death, MM is still an icon, and her estate continues to generate millions of dollars per year. Would this be the case if she had buck teeth or a half-inch gap between her two front teeth...not a chance. Her beauty even overpowered the stigma of mental illness. Let this be a lesson - if you are going to have mental problems, it's better to be pretty and have a nice smile.

As much as I fight it, it's a fact that an attractive smile is important to become a sex symbol in the American society. It's not the only thing that counts but it helps if at least your upper front teeth are reasonably straight and white. It's sometimes odd how some people get focused on some particularly small details in their smile - while ignoring some much bigger issues.

As an example, I was nearing completion of an orthodontic treatment case for a patient who was a teen. He had, much like me at his age, *horrible acne* ...certainly the most distracting feature about him. For some reason he thought one of his teeth was still out of line (and it probably ***was*** about 2 microns off from the others if an electron microscope was used), and although I was tempted to tell him that the truth was NOBODY IN THE WORLD would see past his acne, or notice anything even remotely wrong with the position of the tooth he was obsessing over, I didn't. I didn't tell him the truth because I didn't want to hurt his feelings.

Sometimes the truth is painful. In his case I chose to simply try to tweak his tooth a little, and 'drag out' the treatment in an attempt to 'wear him down', and get him refocused on something else in his life. When you correct one thing, there is often another issue that obsessive personalities latch onto, and the treatment becomes more of a hobby than anything else.

I was well past the stage of trying to make everything perfect, and he had slipped by my personality assessment and managed to get into treatment. One mistake many dentists make is trying to make everyone happy; I would rather cut my losses early and have someone leave my office, than to have a small group of 'pain in the asses' make going to work miserable. The matching of personalities is almost as important as the quality of care, because even if you give someone the best care in the world, and they are not happy, then it is very unsatisfying for everyone involved.

Suzanne Somers is WRONG about Fluoride

The blonde bombshell looks great, thanks to important breakthroughs mentioned in her recent book, and probably more than a couple veneers. Alright, she does look better now than when she had crooked teeth but I would have done something else for her other than porcelain teeth if I had my hands on her first. She may be right about the importance of hormones, but one thing she was <u>wrong</u> about was fluoride. She rambled on about fluoride, which is added to water in many cities to reduce tooth decay, as if it was radioactive. Not that there aren't a few dentists that agree with her, but I think most feel you are better off with fluoride in the water.

The extremely low levels of fluoride added to the water by municipal treatment centers are very beneficial from a dental standpoint. The safety has been studied over the long term, and while high amounts can cause problems, a correct amount is safe. To give you the best review of the subject, we have included a FREE report from an expert in the field, just visit the "*Confessions*" website to get a copy.

REECE "the pug" Witherspoon

This actress has the profile of a pug...and I know pugs, since I have been paying the vet bill for over 8 years on our chubby, bug-eyed lump. I trust that Reece has better breath than our pug, but there is a slight resemblance. The actress appears to have a huge lower jaw, but in fact has what's called in the dental biz - a "mid-face deficiency". This means Reece has a maxilla (upper jaw in layman's terms), which is further back than it should be, which gives her more of a flatter Asian profile.

Her looks surely would have precluded all the nominations, awards and celebrity if an orthodontist would have been on the board. In reality, outside the orthodontist's critical analysis, Reece is an attractive young star who has managed to gain star status - in spite of what an average orthodontist and oral surgeon would have fantasized about with braces, facial bone relocation surgery, and more braces after that. Doing it now would make her nearly unrecognizable, and would depreciate her future value.

Don't Take Cosmetic Dentistry Tips from 'The Real Housewives'!

I know they are sometimes fun to watch, but once the spoiled "housewives" or 'bloodsuckers' as they are sometimes called, start having cosmetic dentistry parties, it's time to change the channel. You can be assured they will be giving you dangerous and incorrect advice, thanks to misinformation provided by a cosmetic dentist anxious to get some television exposure. Properly performed, cosmetic dentistry can't always fit into one episode of a television program.

Many of 'The Real Housewives' are examples of what women become - when they have nothing better to do than 'burn up' money, and to redo everything they possibly can. Eventually they are merely gruesome caricatures of their former selves. HD television sure exposes much of what we didn't really want to see…when do we get to go back to Low Definition?

FACTOID: Without even sleeping with her, my guess would be Bethenny Frankel (Cast, The Real Housewives Of New York City & author of Naturally Thin: Unleash Your SkinnyGirl & Free Yourself from a Lifetime of Dieting) grinds her teeth like crazy in her sleep. Check out her well-developed masseters (jaw muscles) which could not be this huge without constant gum chewing or lots of grinding at night…of her teeth!

Chapter 9
LIES IN MARKETING & PRIMITIVE DENTAL MUTILATIONS

SMILES in Advertising

Smiles that are used in advertising are commonly so far out of the cosmetic dentist's ideal, that we are almost paralyzed by the sight of them. For some reason the models have significant variations, which could only mean a model was related to the company president, or there was some hanky-panky going on with the marketing executive. Maybe its just because of my cosmetic dental training, I focus on the dental flaws that the public barely even notices.

It becomes obvious that dentists have not used their considerable clout to work their way into consulting positions in the audition process and editing room. How can advertisers have a chance at educating the world about truly beautiful smiles without a dental degree?

One shocking example was a poster in IKEA - which featured one of the designers who had a Swedish name that could not be pronounced by 9.5 out of 10 Americans. She had the audacity to smile in a huge poster when she knew dentists would gather and chant in protest. God Bless her for her that.

Success and Your Smile

As discussed, most mega-stars in the movie industry have short comings from a cosmetic dentist's perspective - which make dentists scratch their heads in disbelief. How, we ask ourselves, could they be loved by millions and be paid as much, when their teeth have obvious flaws or they would even be candidates for jaw surgery?

The cosmetic dental societies need to understand the importance of personal motivation and drive as primary forces in a person's success. While cosmetic dentistry and orthodontics can form an important component in helping a person be all they can be, the treatment is seldom the primary reason for a person's well being.

The fact that beautiful people have advantages in society is overshadowed by personal drive, intelligence and ingenuity. Trump would still be as rich if his teeth were not crowned. Bill Gates would still have made billions with an even deeper overbite. Even in the 'pretty people' business, a natural smile will usually be more desirable than one that has been overly altered in the name of scientific perfection.

Taking a phrase from the Obama teleprompter, and giving it a little dental twist…"you can put Veneers on a Pig, but it's still a Pig". If I may be a little cruel, if you look in the mirror and are attractive when you are not smiling, your investment in cosmetic dentistry may be worth it. If what you see in the mirror is not flattering when you are not showing your teeth, then you may need more than cosmetic dentistry.

TRUE/FALSE:
Some Dentists try to correct wrinkles with new teeth.

Answer: There are some dentists who attempt to treat people with wrinkles by over-building a patient's teeth. If your teeth are severely worn down, then this may be an idea. If you have dentures, you may need a new set to compensate for the bone loss that always occurs when teeth are extracted. My suggestion is, if your teeth are fine, skip the dental work and go get a second facelift if it's the wrinkles that are the problem. The face lift will probably be $20,000 cheaper and make a greater improvement.

The Mona Lisa Smile

The most famous smile in the world belongs to the lady in Leonardo da Vinci's portrait called the Mona Lisa. It was painted in the early 1500's, and has survived being stolen by an employee of the Louvre, been doused with acid, and even hit by a rock thrown by a lunatic. Maybe she had a bigger smile before all this abuse. She even had to go into hiding during a World War or two. It's been cleaned, touched up and fumigated more times than Joan Rivers' panty drawer, but she still looks pretty good.

Now Mona isn't really Mona…she's Lisa. Mona came from *ma donna* which meant "my lady"…Monna for short in Italian. She is believed to be the painting of the wife of a wealthy silk merchant from Florence and Tuscany. Curious how it was finally in the hands of the painter's assistant after Leonardo died in 1525. You'd think the picture would have stayed in the merchant's home and been passed down. Maybe he painted a more flattering portrait and this one was returned for store credit.

The funny thing about Mona is her smile…and her plucked eyebrows are a little odd too. Her smile would not reveal enough to capture the attention of the dental community, and yet it has captured the fascination of the rest of the world. Actually, trying to paint and sculpt teeth is quite difficult, and many times the attempts look more like the raking incisors of a Brontosaurus (now called an Apatosaurus)…either way, Leonardo was not stupid. He would leave the dental profession to fight over the definition of a perfect smile which still remains a mystery to this day.

Cosmetic Dentistry through the Ages

The United States has the most unrealistic ideals for dental cosmetics in the world. Teeth tend to be chalky white, big and level, and straight. The over-treated smiles of Liberace and Las Vegas casino owners come to mind as examples. It is like painting flames on the front of a brand new Lamborghini…there is a point where too much is too much. Just because you have the money doesn't mean you need to wear it on your front teeth!

That opens the door to the smiles of the current 'rap' generation. "Pimping Your Smile" means cramming as many fake diamonds and as much platinum and silver jewelry as you can into your 'grill'. While it may be fun for Halloween and MTV awards, it is not healthy. There can be actual harm caused by 'dental bling', and hopefully most participants are smart enough not to wear them more than a few hours at a time.

England has been known for low dental standards due to their budget level dental care system, and "English Teeth" is synonymous with a severely crooked and stained dentition. Their dental health care program attends to the bare essentials, and perhaps luckily for them, only recently has the excitement of cosmetic dentistry seemed to catch fire.

Canada is probably somewhere between these two extremes…and many television personalities seem to slip past the dental censors with smiles resembling Austin Powers. American networks seem to steal any Canadian hosts and personalities that have anything close to a normal smile.

Lip rings and tongue posts have also crept into the smiles and mouths of our youth. They are usually installed by people who are not trained in surgery, who cannot write prescriptions to treat infections, and whose sterilization equipment many have been found in the garage of a deceased dentist or picked up at an estate auction. While they certainly are topics of conversation and can help give the person a degree of separation from their parents, the problems associated with them are numerous.

Lip rings can rub against the gum line and strip the tissue off the teeth. This exposes the root, which can be sensitive and more likely to decay. Tongue rings can lead to broken teeth if the ends are metal, but in a few cases they can lead to infections, 'difficult to control' bleeding, and even death. Why someone is allowed to 'skewer' humans without advanced medical training, while a dental assistant needs to have a certificate to take a mould of your teeth, I will never fully understand.

Russia and Mexico are known for their gold restorations, even in the front teeth. France is known for its love of high fashion and the best things in life, while not so much for concern over mild to moderate amounts of crowding in the dentition.

Going back into history and anthropologic essays by long dead scholars, we find stories of "horrific dental mutilation", which actually may be more conservative than some of the dental care that is done today in the name of smile enhancement. Pound for pound when you compare the actual loss of enamel, dentin, nerve, gum and bone between a person who had a front tooth removed as part of a tribal tradition inside a mud hut, or a patient who has been drilled down for porcelain crowns from ear to ear, there is a big question about which procedure is more barbaric! I would prefer to be lying with my back in the dirt, perhaps partly hypnotized from the effects of a herbal and fermented beverage, than the modern alternative. The slick and supple vinyl and padded headrests, and all the freezing in the world, would never get me interested in a full veneer makeover simply as a cure to straighten my teeth.

Many ancient cultures had specific dental rituals which marked them as members of a tribe, and celebrated their acceptance into adulthood. A brief review may be of interest to some who are still reading, and are not off quivering in a corner. This is not meant to scare you off from dental treatment...I am just trying to temper your enthusiasm until you know the whole story.

According to Humphrey Humphries who presented a lecture back in 1954 titled "Dental Operations Practiced in Primitive Communities", there was dentistry before there were dental schools. Dr. 'Hump' explained that, like today, many dental procedures were performed in ancient societies for ritual or cosmetic purposes and were not therapeutic.

He wrote: "The commonest operation of all is the extraction of front teeth, but it is seldom, if ever, performed on account of caries (decay). Dental caries is as old as *homo sapiens* - even older for it is found not only in his predecessor Neanderthal man, but in 2% of wild monkeys. But with uncivilized peoples, ancient or modern, or in other animal species, it rarely affects the front teeth and mainly attacks the premolars and molars. In the great majority of the cases, primitive tooth extraction is performed on the incisor teeth as one of the initiation ceremonies performed at puberty."

Dr. "H" also mentions this selective extraction procedure was performed by many groups since the last Ice Age, at a time when you didn't have to go to the 7-Eleven to have a yellow colored ice/snow drink. This 'Big Gulp' was yours for the taking with refreshing flavors including mammoth, musk ox and Uncle Harry.

The ritualistic removal of teeth was practiced all over the world, including Africa south of the Sahara, Australia and the Pacific islands including Tasmania, the East Indies and the Philippines. His article suggests some association with certain races, and seems to blame them for spreading the practice to other unrelated groups like the Australian aborigines. At the time he wrote his article in the early 1950's, he stated the selected 'tooth-removal' thing was carried out on boys and girls about the age of 12, which was the usual age of the onset of puberty. This is unlike today where if you don't have a moustache in third grade, you are considered a wimp...or if you are a grade 5 girl without a drawer dedicated to the latest Victoria Secret Spring Collection, you have no friends.

While most tribes engaged in the practice of removing just one upper front tooth, some bucked the tread, so to speak, and extracted 2-4 lower incisors and sometimes the lower canines. He stated this was a feature of the Bangoro tribe of Uganda (or at least the characteristic of the gal he met in the gentleman's club while he was there on safari). The motives for these rituals eluded the researcher, but he explained that like his "today", and like our today about 60 years later, that "It is sufficient for the boys and girls to undergo it, that is, a universal fashion and that if they evade it they will always be conspicuous and a butt for the ridicule of the majority" (or at least with the humanoids with whom they like to "chill out").

He also stated some words that continue to ring true with the following eloquence: "When we witness the much more expensive and equally exhausting ordeals to which modern women subject themselves, so that their hair, their eyebrows, or their finger-nails may be changed from their natural colors and forms to those demanded by the fashion of the day, we can readily understand the tyranny of custom over the small societies of primitive man. Nevertheless, we can perhaps divine something of the motives which lead to the adoption of this painful and - to our eyes - disfiguring rite." Hopefully he hasn't lived to see the excruciating ritual involved in Brazilian bikini waxing...and to think some people are still afraid of the dentist.

Dr. Humphreys continued with explanations about mankind's addiction to sacrifices, including one tribe in Africa that used to cut off the tip of a finger. This idea goes back a long way as cave paintings seem to suggest they did it too. There is also a sickening practice which may even be practiced in some areas today, where newborns males are held down without consent or legal representation, and cut "down there"... sometimes called a "circum-stitch-em" ritual. If you are a newborn reading this as you wait for the guy with the curly sideburns to get to you…jump off the table and make a run for it! If we can save just one of you from this, it will all be worth it.

He mentions some tribes like the Masai in East Africa do a 'double-whammy' and pull a baby front tooth at about 8 months, and the permanent one at about age 12. Something like this is still recommended by some orthodontists today, but I'm in so much trouble already, I'm not going to touch that one.

In an odd practice noted back in 1868, a particular group removed four lower front teeth - reportedly to allow them to lisp properly. Apparently their language when spoken properly involved some serious lisping. A speech therapist would be boiled alive in those days. The Masai justified their upper tooth extraction as a way to allow feeding of those afflicted with lock-jaw, which was common there.

A tribe in Australia (or at least one of the members who was forced to learn English), explained their similar practice was done to boys and girls before marriage so that their smile looked a little more like a particular rain cloud. What they were smoking or drinking at the time they thought this one up was not known. The Oyakumbi tribe of Central Africa had the lower middle two teeth removed, and the upper front ones filed down unless they were part of the royal family - who did not do any dental mutilation (this seems completely opposite to the Royals in the UK who seem to have their teeth made as unsightly as possible). The African tribe justified the practice by saying, with the help of an interpreter, that it made their subjects look like the cattle they owned - since apparently cattle lack the same teeth.

The description of the procedures used in these rituals may be too graphic for some readers. If you start to feel weak, lay down on the floor with your feet up on a chair and keep reading…this is the good part.

The doctor explained that in both the African and Australian tribes, the victim/patient laid on the ground on his/her "back with the head in between the knees or in the lap of the squatting surgeon". While little progress has been made in positioning, at least now the surgeon accepts most credit cards and has staff to help process your insurance forms. True progress has been made in the type of tools or instruments used, as the primitive groups resorted to the use of a stick against the tooth, and a stone to tap the other end. Modern dental surgeons use metal versions of the same design, which allow them to hold up to the sterilization process and not waste time looking for proper sticks and stones.

A forceful blow is a bit of a gamble…if the tribal dentist gives it a good whack, the tooth may fly out or it may just break off at the gum line. Being a dentist, I can sympathize with the hollow sick feeling when your enthusiasm to pull a tooth exceeds the strength of the root. If this was done in front of a group of fellow tribesman, it must have been stressful.

To play it safe, the tribal 'doc' would often start out with a series of moderate taps, and then once it was loose enough, he would use his fingers. Some tribes were able to use scrap metal, perhaps scavenged from English or Dutch explorers who were gored to death by hippos while painting beside a majestic river, or traded for 'a brief fling in a stick hut' with the pretty girl in the tribe.

If the tribe got their hands on metal, they sometimes used another technique. In the case of the Bakitara tribe of Central Africa they had the practice of removing the six lower front teeth at puberty.

Anyway, this tribe had a better budget, and had a dental assistant who held the "patient's" arms and legs with his own, while the main man with the fancy degree "levers out the teeth one by one with a pointed peg of iron six inches long, which he drives down between the gum and the tooth." I know, you're thinking "where do I sign up?", but by now most of these tribal 'docs' are likely selling fake Rolex's in front of the Century 21 store - across from the former Trade Center area in NYC.

This front end work was for cosmetic reasons, while the backend stuff (working on the molars) was generally for dealing with toothache issues. Now I've heard reports, and hopefully they are exaggerated, but if it's true it's as sad as all this African stuff. Apparently, some very desperate models or "wanna-bees" found a dentist just as stupid, who actually pulls out their upper back teeth to give them a sunken-in look to accentuate the cheek bones. This is as stupid as anything I've ever heard of…don't they know that there is a now a lipo-suction procedure for this?

Back to the gore in other cultures…OK, so they use sticks, stones and fingers, but they also occasionally used sinew to pull teeth. We should pause and remind you not to try any of this yourself at home, unless of course you have exceeded your yearly maximum on your dental plan.

The detailed report goes on to describe some odd rituals which follow the extraction ...*well not as weird as putting a baby tooth under a kid's pillow and telling him/her that a little fairy is going to replace it with money while they sleep.* Now that's a parent that is either not taking medication on time or has some serious delusions...at this very moment in a hut in Africa, tribespeople are reading about this common practice in the USA and thinking "WTH"?

Some of the tribes of Central Australia took the extracted tooth involved in the ritual, and threw it as far as possible. Other times the tooth was pounded into a powder, and eaten by some very special people. The lucky tooth eaters were the mom if it was the daughter, and the mother-in-law if a boy was the victim. Other tribes buried the tooth beside the water hole to inspire the rain gods.

The shape of teeth was routinely altered by certain tribes. "Perhaps the simplest mutilation was that of grinding down the teeth with stone till a space appeared between the upper and lower incisor edges." Of course, modern dentists and orthodontists still do this today, but we struggle with trying to find an insurance code to pay for it.

Another form of tooth mutilation performed in the Philippines and in Central America was the shaping of the front teeth into a point. Sometimes the teeth were ground in a way which made them have multiple points for each tooth "to resemble the teeth of a comb".

In a fascinating and detailed description which we will repeat here... "the appearance of the teeth is sometimes changed without alteration of their shape by coating them with some artificial application. Some tribes in New Guinea and the Philippines Islands cover their teeth with black lacquer prepared by mixing a soil containing sulphur with a pungent leaf: they have to abstain from eating and talking for several days while the lacquer hardens. Marco Polo records that in the thirteenth century wealthy Chinese sometimes covered their teeth with thin plates of gold, an anticipation of jacket crowns".

Dr. 'Hump' was most impressed with the dental work of the pre-Columbian people of South America, and their expert ability at inserting precious stones into the front teeth. "In the great majority of cases these were green-jade, jadeite or turquoise -though rock crystal and obsidian have been recorded." He also mentioned head hunters in the Philippines had crude inlays in their front teeth.

A few years ago it was common in North America to have patients request diamonds or simulated stones to be inserted into their front teeth. A small hole was drilled, and it was held in with bonding. Wow, we've come a long way, baby!

Back in ancient SA, "the art (of tooth jewels) was imitated by the neighbors of the Maya to the South as well as in Mexico, for it has been recorded from Ecuador where in one case the inlay was gold." As in the case of cosmetic crowns and veneers today, the ornamentation which involved drilling into the teeth sometimes resulted in the death of the nerve of the tooth - and lead to an abscess. The type of cement used to make the gems stick eluded their investigations, but it's safe to say it was their own version of Crazy Glue®.

While it was unlikely to be just an ornamental event, several cultures invented the concept of using gold wire twisted around teeth that presumably were a little loose, due to gum disease that spread into the bone. The practice occurred in both South America and in Italy, where the Etruscans used the technique as early as the seventh century B.C. The early Italians experimented with cast gold, and replacing missing teeth with fake ones carved from ox teeth. They shared their skills with other civilizations in the trading area.

Many early societies dealt with dental issues outside the cosmetic concerns, and some fascinating descriptions included the following:

"Australian aborigines will heat the pointed end of a stick in the fire and thrust it into the cavity. The Moros of Liberia fill it with country salt (potassium hydroxide) or red pepper seeds, either of which, like arsenic, produces death of the pulp (nerve) and stops the pain. Many savages employ toothpicks, or brush their teeth with green sticks frayed at the end. This is still the standard toothbrush in India, a very efficient one which I have myself used on active service. Today (1954) with increasing European contact, most of the operations I have described are becoming obsolescent."

The primitive dental mutilations in the name of beauty have been replaced by something that seems equally odd …what dentists do now with *extreme smile makeovers.*

What the heck is a Smile Anyway?

To be frank with you, the whole concept of a smile has become screwed up. Dental school has taught dentists how to repair teeth, but courses after that have distorted their perceptions. Most dentists consider a smile the part of a person that shows when the lips are stretched back over a person's face. We pull back your lips with what seems to be modified retractors invented by gynecologists (oooh, that's cold!), and want to see you up close.

Unless you're Mick Jagger or Steven Tyler, use lots of lip balm for the few weeks before your dentist photo shoot this is going to be a bit of a stretch. The dentist's cameras have fancy ring flashes that besides causing temporary blindness capture every little crack, chip, twist and turn, space and stain…things nobody else has ever noticed about you.

Then just when you think they are done, the assistant pulls out the *sigmoid-o-scope,* borrowed from the proctologist still dripping with disinfectant. She "takes the tour" around your orifice and snaps pictures of the ugliest things she can find…kind of like the Paparazzi getting photographs of Hollywood stars without makeup and eating chili dogs.

Then, if that's not enough, they put the pictures up on a screen and everyone who walks by stops and gasps in horror. The dentist is called in with a code red…lucky you. The doc straps on his microscope to his eyewear and plugs in a headlamp. You start to wonder if they will appraise your jewels as part of the deal, but you are too embarrassed to ask.

The dentist reads off a bunch of numbers and words that can't mean anything in English. He says the number 13 with a mesio-bucco-distal-occlusal-lingual…you think "Gawd doc…how long do I have to live?" The gibberish continues and then you think you hear the dentist mumble "OK…I think that about covers my alimony payment this month."

The doc gets up and explains he has someone who can help you work out the financing and explain things properly. Now, let's stop here and get back to the fact that the doc doesn't even know what a real smile is anymore. Here's why…

A smile is an expression of the whole face and not just the display of enamel which is viewed when you are forced to say "mama". Your eyes can be smiling…you can even smile without teeth! You may start to think who needs a dentist anyway?

You probably know more about a natural smile than your average dentist…you know a smile is a good one when it makes you smile back (or makes you feel obligated to leave a gratuity). You don't need to have a dental degree to recognize a 'hot' smile, and your opinion is just as important as those docs who are accredited members of the AACD. Discuss the things you feel are important with your dentist and if he/she doesn't seem to get it, then seek a second opinion.

Hypnotized Dentists at War

As silly as it sounds dental professionals are constantly forming groups, much like the gangs in an LA turf war. Rarely do they venture across into the other gang's zone – fearing they may become indoctrinated into another school of thought. Many of these so-called gangs are funded by dental companies that provide education – to help promote their own products.

The technology available in dentistry is truly astounding, and who would have thought a few years ago that a laser now would be sitting in the corner of many typical dental offices across North America. Captain Kirk would have been impressed if the Starship Enterprise had digital x-rays that instantly appeared on a flat screen, and cosmetic imaging could demonstrate how you may look after a cosmetic smile enhancement. Sometimes the costs are outrageous and many dentists 'get in way over their heads', because they buy more dental toys than they can afford. After a while we grow resentful that the dental equipment sales reps are driving faster cars and taking more holidays than we are.

Technology is great, but the marketplace is extremely competitive. Companies have become very aggressive at signing dentists into their "educational" programs. Dentists are getting used to having to purchase something at almost every convention or seminar they attend. From dental school, they are programmed to sit and listen, ask few questions and regurgitate what the lecturer said on the examination. If you questioned the rules you didn't pass. Unfortunately the universities do not have the budgets to continue the educational process, and they leave it up to the private sector to add more skills to the dentists after graduation.

So the doctors are primed and easy targets for the savvy companies that try to get their business. The exotic locations and hotels lure the dentists, but the bottom line is *they want to sell things for the dentist to put in your mouth, whether or not it is the best thing for you*.

This is not really a bad thing if the product is as useful as it claims. It's kind of like having that nice aunt come over for dinner, and then, at the end of the night you are signed up for a garage full of Amway products. There is a dentist advocate group that independently tests assorted dental products called the Clinicians Report, but many dentists do not adequately research the things they buy, which may put patients at risk.

It is not only the manufacturing companies that participate in this game of grabbing the dentists' wallets; dental laboratories don't sit back and hope for business. *Dental labs have become very assertive and try to pick up on controlling a dentist's education where dental school left off.* Unfortunately, their goal is to get the doc hypnotized to sell more of their lab work to the consumer. The programs are polished very well, and sneak up on the poor unsuspecting dentist. If the course is on Friday they hope the dentist is already trying to offer the procedure to you on Monday morning.

In fact, many dental association meetings which you would expect to be offered by independent researchers from universities are actually sponsored by dental manufacturers and dental labs. *In short, the dental training is corrupted by free enterprise and is not nearly as clean as you would expect*. Even universities, which are underfunded by the government, are forced to accept money from outside parties with ulterior motives, specifically wanting to plug their own products and advertise any tests that show they are superior to other brands.

While dentistry would still be in the stone ages if it wasn't for these labs and profit-driven companies, both dentists and patients need to be aware of these forces. Once a dentist becomes part of a program, it usually is a series which over the years makes the doctor little more than a 'drone' - sapping his/her ability to think independently.

As far as being at war, sometimes these groups form widely separated beliefs or philosophies that totally contradict each other. Each side thinks the other is crazy. If they get into the same room, some of these individuals actually become very hostile, and it's surprising few dentists have been physically injured. If the odd individual ever crosses party boundaries, it is considered a major coup, and much gloating and 'chest banging' can be heard.

In 1833, back when Andrew Jackson was president of the United States, there was a huge war among dentists, which threatened the profession. It was about the new silver-mercury filling material that was just invented. Many believed the filling to be hazardous and that it didn't work, but it caught on and still serves to this day probably even in Oprah's mouth. While most studies show it is safe, it is now rarely used due to the improvements in white fillings.

With present day in-fighting within the profession, the amalgam issue is still debated, and another battle relates to where people's perfect bite should be. As silly as it sounds, dentists can't even agree on the right place to bite! There is also disagreement related to different styles of orthodontic treatment (tooth straightening).

The assorted beliefs that dental professionals have are so ingrained from intense training experiences, that they sometimes have the intensity of a religious fanatic. I've been attacked many times about my own thoughts and enjoy retaliating as much as anyone. Try converting a devout Catholic to Muslimism, or a Jew to Buddhism, and you'll know what I'm talking about. It gets pretty ugly, and there have been incidents of slander and threats. It's as if one insulted the other guy's mother. While Jerry Springer would smile with glee at some of the antics, it is somewhat embarrassing to see professionals act this way.

In the end, all this in-fighting is a good thing and the overall winner is the patient. <u>The wars over the right way to do things reveal the truth that there is in fact no universally accepted standard of care for anything we do in dentistry</u>. The slight variations that we fight over may only be measured in millimeters, but that's the level at which most dentists think. The fact is a 2-3 millimeter difference can sometimes mean a $30-50,000 difference in your dental bill depending on the philosophy of the dental professional!

This is a very important concept that most people are totally in the dark about…the beliefs that the individual dental professional has can cost you dearly (and we are not just talking about money).

Chapter 10
GUMS, YOUR KID'S UGLY SMILE & AVOIDING OLD-FASHIONED ORTHODONTISTS: LET'S TALK OFF THE RECORD.

Gum Disease Can Give You an UGLY Smile

How your teeth look is also determined by your gums. In a recent publication the following thoughts were mentioned:

"According to the currently accepted theory of the development of periodontal disease, known as the specific plaque hypothesis, only a limited group of bacteria has the capacity to cause periodontitis (gum disease that eats away the bone around your teeth). The occurrence of the infection depends on there being a sufficient concentration of the periodontal pathogens and these pathogens must express virulence factors. A person can harbor these pathogens without presenting any clinical symptoms. Symptoms appear only if the host's defense mechanisms are no longer able to maintain a healthy (balance), and the host's immune response modulates disease progression towards destruction.

Mechanical debridement of the dental biofilm and elimination of the local irritating factors are the basis of periodontal therapy, but are not effective for all sites and forms of periodontal disease. The use of antibiotics is warranted for certain patients. Systemically administered antibiotics can reach micro-organisms that are inaccessible to scaling instruments. However, in deciding whether to use curative systemic antibiotics, it is important to consider the potential benefits and adverse effects, including the development of resistant bacterial species."

What this means in English is that it's smart to get your teeth professionally cleaned regularly, and sometimes the dentist will need to give you a prescription. There are some new things including laser treatment and even gels that you can wear in special trays to kill off the bacteria that live around your teeth. It is like trying to get rid of cockroaches...they 'breed like hell', and unless you keep killing them off your mouth will become infested again.

Gum disease can loosen your teeth and cause spaces, even leading to buck teeth, and eventually tooth loss. Smokers and diabetics are at higher risk of suffering from this problem. So if you are over-due for a cleaning, call your dentist today. DentistryForDiabetics.com may have some additional information on this topic.

You DON'T Always Need to Replace Lost Teeth

Contrary to what most dentists say, you don't always need to replace a missing tooth. Most people can chew with only half their teeth, and if you lose a tooth at the very back of your mouth you may be fine without it. When a tooth is lost in the middle, the others often tip into the space or grow down if the opposing one has nothing to bite against; so discuss the consequences of any lost tooth with your dentist, and ask whether or not it should be replaced. If your brushing and flossing abilities are below average, you may be better off not replacing any missing teeth until your hygienist gives you two thumbs up, or if she is very picky one thumb and a pinky.

The Cost of Perfection

In nature, the world is not perfect. The most beautiful people on earth have flaws, so why all the fuss? Very few of the cosmetic parameters need to be 100% perfect to be perfectly acceptable and this is my point to any dentist reading this short story. A nice smile has some irregularities that do not need to be treated. Accepting some irregularities as a patient will likely save you thousands of dollars, and actually reduce your risk of complications.

Cosmetic dentistry, along with the obvious benefits, can also cause harm. The less treatment you need the better. If you can get by with less treatment, any more will add to the risk of complications.

A dentist with more experience and skill will generally have a lower complication risk. Even if the results are excellent and no complications are experienced, as time goes by, dental work will need replacement. Whether it is 7 or 12 years, the cost of replacing the restorations in the future will be even more substantial and carry another exposure to risks, perhaps even greater than at the first experience.

Problems with Orthodontic Practitioners

I've 'dumped' on the cosmetic dentists enough, so now I will turn my near-sighted, critical eye to the dental professionals who straighten teeth with wires and appliances. As a group they probably cause less damage to teeth than their "cosmetic" colleagues, but some of them are out of touch with reality. Some of the concerns that have been raised about Orthodontists include:

1. They charge too much for simple things and not enough for complicated cases.

2. They take too long and waste time on small details.

3. They are sometimes rude to other dental professionals who offer braces.

4. They each think their way of straightening teeth is the only way.

5. They haven't stood up and told the public that cosmetic dentists shouldn't be straightening healthy teeth with veneers.

6. They have hidden information from the public about risks involved in longer orthodontic treatment times.

7. They don't always refer back to the dentist who sent them the patient in the first place, and sometimes they do not ask the regular dentist for input regarding the treatment during the process.

Orthodontists have their own set of high standards and are extremely fussy. Different groups of orthodontists have totally different standards, so there is always controversy even within the orthodontic community. This desire to meet specific ideals may get in the way of the fact that their customers don't like wearing braces for the years they are often needed, and forces some people to become victims of "instant orthodontics" (veneers) at the hands of the cosmetic dentists. I think there is still hope for orthodontists, and actually think they will soon be busier than ever when patients know more about the new kinds of braces that are available.

Common Mistakes Your Family Dentist may make that can affect Orthodontic Treatment

Probably the biggest problem is the general dentist may miss an orthodontic problem in a child that could be corrected easier when it is first identified. Adults often have significant orthodontic or cosmetic issues that general dentists can miss during routine examinations. A complaint orthodontists have is some general dentists "dabble" in orthodontics and may take on cases that exceed their skill level. If a dentist wants to offer orthodontics he will need to make a large commitment to additional education and do more than a couple weekend courses.

The thing that irritates me, and likely other dental professionals that provide orthodontics, is the dentist who goes ahead with crown and bridge work before being sure the patient could not be helped with some orthodontic tooth movement first. It's also important to evaluate whether or not a major change in the bite position may be needed prior to doing even one simple crown (as in the situation where people have moderate to severe wear on their teeth).

Once crowns are placed over the teeth it is tougher to attach the brackets onto the porcelain without risking damage to the new crown. Crowns, like veneers are sometimes used to "straighten" teeth and this also makes orthodontics more complicated. *In fact, it is then necessary to cut off the crowns and bridges and place temporary crowns on the teeth back into the "crooked" positions, so the teeth can be aligned properly before doing the crowns/bridgework all over again.*

As you can probably, tell this "back-tracking" adds additional expense and it can add thousands of dollars to the dentist's pockets that you'd otherwise be able to blow on other things. So if you are being told you need a crown, or a bridge, be sure to ask if orthodontics may be required. Even if you have had a root canal done in a back tooth, it can be filled in such a way to protect it until after the orthodontics are completed.

Treating Severely Worn Teeth with Braces & Bonding?

As mentioned people who have very worn teeth can be a challenge. They usually need the expertise of dental professionals trained in cosmetics, reconstruction and orthodontics. Commonly a general dentist will make the mistake of fixing single problems without regard for the whole mouth. For example, a chipped tooth may be capped into the "old worn down" position, and is a compete waste of money if the person needs to have all the teeth built up again. Sometimes orthodontic treatment is needed to help position the teeth after the worn areas are replaced with composite or temporary crowns. I'd suggest asking the dentist to use composite material wherever possible, so that you do not have a mouth full of acrylic temporaries.

Dentists who have taken courses from the Spear Institute or Dr. John Kois have additional training that would aid in treating this type of situation. Alternatively, a prosthodontic specialist would also be able to provide guidance for a patient with this complex problem. The prosthodontist (instead of the general dentist) would usually take the lead role in being the "general contractor" and would coordinate all the treatment with other practitioners as needed. Specialists tend to prefer working with other specialists, so if orthodontics is needed in combination with the re-tipping of the teeth, an orthodontist may be called in to help on the project.

FACTOID: Bruxism or tooth grinding is extremely destructive to teeth and even the most expensive cosmetic makeover can be shattered to bits. Your dentist may prefer to move or retire rather than to warranty the work if you are a heavy grinder. Many patients say "I don't grind my teeth", but they also say they don't snore or pass gas. Wearing a special night guard will be the best investment you can make.

What Your "ORTHODENTIST" Doesn't Want You to Know About Aligners – as critiqued by an Aligner Expert

Straightening teeth with orthodontic braces has come a long way since the days of headgear/straps and silver bands and painfully stiff wires. As far as we have come, there is still a long way to go before we meet the needs of the public for a fast and affordable alternative to traditional braces. There are some people that don't want to wear braces, so they try plastic aligners instead.

Invisalign® is the best known brand of orthodontic appliances that uses a series of clear aligners to make small movements in the teeth. Behind all the fancy advertisements and the promise of straighter teeth without braces, aligners work well for very simple orthodontic problems, but are thought by many to be not as great for complex situations. If the dentist only knows how to take impressions for aligner trays, and is not experienced with using braces, you may be in for trouble.

Many times the dental professional will try to treat a situation which is simply too difficult for aligners, and then after a year or two the patient will need to have braces anyway. If he/she doesn't know how to use braces, then you may need to fight about who is going to pay for the next phase of treatment. For this reason I'd recommend only doing aligner treatment with a dental professional who is also trained in orthodontic care. In fact, if both braces and aligners need to be used, it is usually better to start with the braces and finish the last minute changes with the aligners.

Aligner courses make it seem like the dentist can simply take a few impressions and sit back and hand out a few trays every month or so. It takes much of the thought process out of the doctor's hands, and lets the lab company do all the work. The system didn't work quite as well as it was originally designed, so now little attachments on the teeth are sometimes needed. Another problem is that people don't always wear their aligners enough, and so the time needed is usually much longer than expected.

The cost of aligner treatment is often more than braces, and there is no guarantee that you will not need to wear braces too - so the dental professional may need to factor that cost into the estimate too. Even with the technical problems involved in this option, aligners are a better choice for treating crooked teeth when compared to the alternative of doing porcelain veneers on healthy, good looking teeth. A final thought is that if you are interested in this treatment concept, it may be best to find someone who has performed a large number of cases using aligners, or ask for a special price if a dental professional is using you as a test subject.

CRITIQUE: *"I do think that Invisalign® can treat some tough cases, BUT the dental professional has to have an orthodontic background. Check out some of our cases and you will see tough cases can be done with aligners. Without significant orthodontic training, the dentist must relinquish the planning of the case to the technician and often movements are designed into the case that won't happen in reality. This will lead to poor results. So to sum up, I would agree that a patient needs to choose an experienced dentist or orthodontist whether they want aligners or braces, and should know the pros and cons of each ahead of time."*

Declan J. Devereux, D.D.S.
Visit us online at www.drdeclan.com

*Invisalign® is a registered trademark of align technology – visit Invisalign.com for further information.

Self-Esteem & Your Child's Teeth

In a recent scientific study in orthodontics, the effect of an ugly smile on children with good self-esteem and poor self-esteem was evaluated. The kids were rated from one to four by the official Dental Ugliness Rating Scale.

The research found that kids with healthy self-esteem were not significantly affected by having an unattractive smile. They were less self-conscious of their hideous smiles than those children with low self-esteem.

It could be concluded that kids with good self-esteem would be less likely to be motivated to wear braces. Therefore, for an orthodontist, it is very important to either find a child who is psychologically weakened and looks to the dentist to help them out of their gloom, or find a kid who has a parent who is terrified by their kid's smile (who will willingly pay for the orthodontic braces). <u>Braces appear to be more for the parent's psychological well-being than the child's</u>. The orthodontic profession thrives on the false belief that we need to give our kids perfect smiles.

It may be more important to help these poor kids with self-esteem issues than it is to straighten their crooked teeth.

"Don't make the mistake of feeling like braces for your teenager are more important than a college education…if their smile has a few minor things that they don't seem to care about, they can always pay for it later. The fact is, unless they are extremely motivated to have a new smile they will very likely stop wearing their retainers and within a few years end up with close to the same problem they started with. Only significant orthodontic issues should be considered urgent in the early teens. The dentist and orthodontist can sometimes make you feel like a bad parent if you don't have kids with perfect teeth, but your child's success in life and happiness may not be connected as closely to this as they would be led to believe." – Michael Zuk DDS

TRUE/FALSE:
If you are a senior, you may be too old for braces.

Answer: Actually braces can produce very impressive results for patients of any age and any time you can move a tooth into a better position than "drill it into place" is a smart choice.

Speech Therapy and the Ventriloquist's Dummy

Being a little cynical by nature, I just thought of an analogy that will hurt many therapists' feelings but may have some truth to it. Let's discuss the use of speech therapy, and the relationship with orthodontics. In the last week or two before I wrote this section, a mom came in with her son or daughter and said she had just been to another orthodontic practitioner. She was concerned that the orthodontist wanted her teen to get speech therapy before getting braces…the main concern was that the therapy was going to cost almost as much as the braces. It was also going to take many appointments and many visits that were a substantial investment in time, for both the parent and the teenager.

Some dentists and orthodontists feel speech therapy should form an integral part of the treatment of people who have certain bite issues (usually an open bite - which is where the teeth don't all meet). I have to disagree, and instead agree with one of my orthodontist mentors, that the practice may be mostly a waste of time and money.

I relate this more to someone learning the skills of a being a ventriloquist. Learning to talk without moving your lips, while your hand is stuffed up the rear of a puppet takes serious training.

You can learn to use different parts of your mouth including your tongue, lips, soft palate, uvula (it's not what you're thinking), and directing air through the various structures of your upper airways, to make the same sounds as someone who is missing one of the elements. In the case of the ventriloquist, they are barred from using their lips…if their lips move too much they are not yet a master of the art.

You can likely hire a highly skilled and well-paid therapist, or a dental assistant who took a weekend course, to teach yourself how to talk differently…maybe even swallow differently. I just wonder why you should bother. If your teeth are going to be moved, then you or your child will have to adapt to a new set of circumstances anyway. All I can say is there are differing opinions on the value of speech therapy in the treatment of orthodontic problems.

The BIGGEST Lies in Orthodontics

Orthodontists may not be intentionally lying, but they disagree with each other so much they can't all be right. When I use the term "Orthodontist," I am also referring to general dentists and children's dentists who perform orthodontics and not just certified orthodontic specialists who limit themselves to doing braces. Here are some of the biggest myths that you may hear about orthodontics:

- Early treatment (doing some correction before the teen years) is a waste of time.
- Faster Braces can cause damage to the teeth
- Teeth cannot be moved faster

- You need to correct all the things an orthodontist says are out of line
- Only an Orthodontic specialist knows how to do orthodontic braces
- You need to have all your teeth straightened, not just the front ones
- Orthodontists will wait until just the right time to put braces on your child
- Orthodontists will always use the best braces and wires
- Orthodontists know the right way to straighten teeth
- Speech therapy helps correct orthodontic problems
- Head gear is still needed to treat certain situations
- "Small Jaw" appliances actually help grow the bones.
- Orthodontists know when to start braces when working with an Oral Surgeon who will be needed to reposition the jaw/bones of face
- Orthodontic Specialists are always better at braces than general practitioners and kid's dental specialists (pedodontists)
- You never need to pull teeth before braces
- You always need to pull teeth before braces
- What Specialists learn in Orthodontic School is not also taught to other dental professionals
- There is only one way to straighten teeth properly and Orthodontists all do it the exact same way
- Orthodontists are unhappy when you stop wearing your retainer (if you had your braces done elsewhere).

Let's just review a few of my favorites to elaborate on the orthodontic myths in this section, and discuss others later so you know a little more about the controversy about braces..To start with there is absolutely no universal agreed upon treatment goal for the whole orthodontic profession. <u>In fact, they actually acknowledge the fact that they can't even define what "Straight Teeth" really are</u>! That's interesting isn't it?

Not only do orthodontists not agree on where your teeth should be after you are "done", they don't agree on how to get the job accomplished, and how long it should take. There are some doctors who take years and years to finish orthodontic training, and once you are in treatment it seems like it's a life sentence. Often they are trying to "detail" the position of the teeth so much they lose track of time. They are often doing the last year or two just to be sure you catch up on your payments.

Orthodontic practitioners are sometimes too cheap to buy the best brackets and wires - which can slow your treatment or mean many more appointments than are really necessary. It may also be a mistake to get the "designer" brackets that come in assorted shapes/designs simply as a novelty. They do not come in the style with clasps (little clips, sometimes called self-ligating brackets) and so you are paying a price in time with this novelty idea so you can have a little star or lucky charm on your tooth. <u>Picking colors also means you are getting the cheap brackets with the little elastics that hold the wire in</u>. Simply put - the shorter time you are in braces to get the desired result the better.

QUOTE: *"The general dentist needs to incorporate some orthodontics into his/her practice. Orthodontics is the cornerstone of the cosmetic dental practice." – Dr. G. Christensen, Journal of ADA, Dec. 2006.*

TRUE/FALSE:
Orthodontic wires need to be removed at hygiene appointments.

Answer: While hygienists may throw a tantrum, many top orthodontic practitioners recommend that the wire be left in the brackets during a hygiene visit to reduce the cost involved in multiple orthodontic appointments. The hygienist can clean around the wires and should concentrate more on helping the patient learn how to properly clean around the orthodontic hardware.

Let's share with you something that the orthodontic association does not want you to know…. <u>longer times in braces are now believed</u>

to be linked to a higher risk of root damage (not shorter times as previously thought), and longer times in braces also put you at greater risk of "decalcification" or white spots on your teeth because even 'keeners' have a tough time keeping teeth clean with braces in the way.

There is also a turf war between some orthodontic specialists versus general dentists and pedo-dontists (specialists for kids). While some specialists work together, a number of orthodontic specialists have grown resentful of the fact that others are learning how to perform orthodontics by taking additional courses. Often these courses are taught by the same orthodontic specialists who taught the orthodontic grad students, so the training is usually identical except non-specialists are discouraged from treating advanced cases that involve oral surgery in addition to the braces.

So orthodontists have stood back and watched cosmetic dentists drill away crooked healthy teeth for veneers, but if they start doing braces some orthodontists freak out and are very resentful!!!! I'm talking about the equivalent of a Holy Jihad. This battle has gotten very dirty, but in the end the patients will have more options, and competition keeps the prices from getting out of hand. At least in my geographic area, the cost of braces, even for relatively simple situations, made me shudder, and it was an inspiration to learn how to offer braces so I could treat my own children and other patients under my care.

As probably one of the few cosmetic dentists who retreated from "instant orthodontics" (Instant Ortho was a term for a Veneer makeover), I was able to apply many things learned throughout the cosmetic training that made orthodontics easier and faster. It was also possible to see things differently, and find ways to solve some common cosmetic problems by combining the skills from cosmetic dentistry and orthodontics.

Soon we will share the new advances in orthodontics that make 'fast' braces the best way to treat many of the cosmetic dental problems that exist.

FACTOID: Some leading orthodontic educators question the safety and long term problems that may be associated with popular orthodontic devices such as the 100 year old HERBST Appliance (used to treat "small jaws") and headgear (the head straps that teens are sometimes instructed to wear and don't anyway). Are there alternatives to these appliances? Yes, but many orthodontists cling to the past.

OVERHEARD recently at an Exclusive Orthodontic Meeting:

"If braces take much longer than two years then the patient should have been treated surgically instead."- A Top Orthodontic lecturer.

More things to consider about Traditional Orthodontics

There are a few other "naughty" things that patients are not aware of that could affect their orthodontic treatment:

1. Sometimes braces are put on early to "capture" a patient's business and prevent them from going elsewhere. This forces a child to wear braces longer than they need to just so the orthodontic provider can keep his hands in your wallet.

2. Treatment may be dragged out so the patient gets better insurance coverage.

3. Treatment may be delayed when the patient falls behind on their payments (pre-paying may get you a discount and get your treatment completed sooner!).

4. Missing appointments will delay treatment.

5. Not doing what you are told (like proper use of elastics) will delay treatment.

6. Slow 'old style' brackets are cheaper, so many orthodontists/dentists still use them.

7. Patients sometimes forget about routine dental care during braces, and this can lead to ugly spots and decay (it is doubly important to see the hygienist during orthodontic care).

8. General dentists with cosmetic training and orthodontic training can often provide orthodontics for the average case at a level that is competitive with orthodontists (they usually will refer surgical cases to an orthodontist who will work with an oral surgeon).

9. If an orthodontist is performing the treatment, you should

see your general dentist regularly during treatment to be sure things are progressing how the family dentist feels it should. It is disappointing to think you are done, only to have another practitioner who is involved ask for further tweaking.

*

"Man's mind, stretched to a new idea, never goes back to its original dimensions."
-Oliver Wendell Holmes

*

Retainers and the Secret to keeping your Teeth Straight

Retainers are dental appliances that are used to keep teeth in a particular position, usually after they have been moved with some type of orthodontic procedure. There are a number of retainers to choose from, and some are removable and others are not. The current research suggests that the key to keeping your teeth straight after braces is not related to how long you wore the braces, it's how long you wear your retainers.

The bonded retainers are typically a fitted wire that is glued to the inside of the teeth. It is hidden from sight, and soon it is not even noticeable to your tongue. They are used to keep the lower front teeth straight. Bonded wires can make flossing difficult, and more frequent cleanings are needed. The lingual wire retainer does loosen and fall off on occasion ; therefore, it needs to be monitored by your dentist.

Some people prefer to have removable retainers only, and the Essex retainer and the Holley are the two main types. The Essex retainer is a clear plastic retainer that is vacuum-formed to a model of the teeth. It snaps in, and is typically worn at night after getting braces removed. It is fairly durable, but removing it with undue care can break it.

The Holley retainer is the typical retainer you see on television - with the wire in the front and an acrylic part that fit's the inside of the teeth. It allows the bite to settle, but they are also easily broken or lost. Pets seem to enjoy eating all the removable orthodontic retainers, and they are probably the world's most expensive chew toy. The habit of always keeping your retainer in a protective case with your phone number on it will help solve some of the problems. Since many are also accidentally thrown in the trash when wrapped in napkins at restaurants, you should not keep them on a food tray when you take them out.

FACTOID: Some orthodontists now just recommend wearing retainers at night or at home to reduce the risk of losing them. Too many retainers have been lost at school or left beside plates in restaurants to mention.

If you have the tooth grinding condition called *bruxism*, you will quickly destroy or loosen most types of retainers. You may think that you don't clench or grind your teeth at night, but if your dentist notices a significant amount of wear on your enamel, you probably grind in your sleep. Likely half the population does this, and often we don't know why. Stress, bite irregularities and certain medications can cause this to be a problem. Grinding can actually be extremely harmful to your teeth, and lead to short and stubby teeth, cracked molars and cavities. Decay can start in the micro-cracks that form in the teeth, so this can really ruin a perfect set of teeth.

If your dentist suspects that you are a "bruxer" or grinder, then they should recommend a high performance night guard – which also serves double duty as a retainer. To keep your front teeth straight, you will want to have a guard that covers at least the front six teeth. The super-mini grinding guards, like the NTI® brand, may not be large enough to keep your teeth from shifting.

Special situations may require unconventional retainers. As an example, when a space between the front teeth is closed there is a high risk of rebound or relapse with the space reappearing. If you treat your spaced Schwarzenegger/Letterman smile with braces, your dentist or orthodontist may need to bond them together with a fiber similar to Kevlar. It is usually hidden behind the teeth and designed to flex a little with normal function. Occasionally they may come loose, and you may need to have the space closed again with a little more orthodontics - but if it is caught early it may only take a few weeks. If the teeth are a little narrow the space can also be closed with a composite (tooth-colored restoration) rather than a veneer.

There is new research that suggests that a dental retainer can serve a number of purposes, which all help reduce the need for further dental treatment. A new idea is the concept of using specific gels inside the retainers, which can potentially reduce a patient's risk of tooth decay and gum disease (discussed in more detail on the website). This is especially exciting news to people that dislike getting dental work!

When ALL you have is a HAMMER... everything looks like a NAIL

Cosmetic dentists usually find a way to treat aesthetic problems with veneers. Orthodontists treat cosmetic problems with orthodontic braces. In a perfect world they would work together and give patients a superior result because usually there are problems that are best treated by a little help from each side. In the real world, these groups rarely work well together.

The cosmetic dentist will often say to a patient, "You could treat this with braces for 2-3 years, or we could get you done in two or three appointments." This has been a pretty easy sale, unless the patient has read this book and understands the shortcomings of veneering. A few years ago, in my ignorance I ran a cosmetic dentistry radio ad that put down the option of orthodontics. The ad brought in loads of people who were all interested in a quick cosmetic fix. I saw some people who would benefit from veneers, but many more that would be better off with braces instead. It wasn't rocket science to see the enormous potential that a faster orthodontic program would have. People wanted straight teeth but they didn't want to wear braces for years and years.

I made a choice to learn orthodontics and other straightening techniques, and was then able to offer either veneers, aligners, orthodontics or a combination, depending on what I thought was best (and not by what my previous limitations were). When I combined everything I learned about cosmetic dentistry, together with the fastest technologies in orthodontics, the result was a service that was competitive with the individual choices of a veneer makeover, traditional braces and aligners.

QUOTE from a respected authority on esthetic & restorative dentistry:

"Whenever applicable, I always advise patients with the option of orthodontic treatment as a substitute for extensive veneer treatment if it makes the final result less invasive."

Chapter 11
CHAPTER 11 FOR THE 'VENEER' NAZIS? ….OMINOUS THOUGHT!

What's the Alternative?

You had to know we had an answer for you…it's the most underused dental service available to patients who want a nicer smile. It's rapid or shorter term orthodontics…a type of braces/cosmetic dentistry combo. We don't use the old fashioned slow poke braces technique, but instead a new brand called High Speed Braces®. Speed is a relative thing and if something can be corrected in 2 years rather than four, or three months rather than nine without significant compromise then it may be worth considering.

Orthodontics has been called the cornerstone of the cosmetic dentistry, but in the age of porcelain veneer makeovers, this essential building block has been left out - making the massive empire of cosmetic dentistry at risk of tumbling, unless drastic steps are taken now. The prediction I am making is that very shortly, the cosmetic revolution will topple, and many "aggressive" cosmetic dentists will be in serious trouble if the members do not wake up soon, re-train and learn to use faster orthodontic braces in combination with the least amount of veneer treatment - as a way to treat patients more conservatively and affordably.

Another Dentist Agrees:

This is an amazing time in dentistry. It is now possible, in just a few months, to achieve an extreme smile makeover *with your own teeth, without having to grind them down..*

I get very passionate about High Speed Braces™ when I tell my patients that I can offer them 80% improvement in the appearance of their smile in about 20% of the time it would take for conventional orthodontics.

And that last 20% improvement is imperceptible to the untrained eye! It's arduous to achieve, and lost extremely quickly when retention is not adhered to religiously! When my patients are shown the evidence of this, they hop on board the HSB bandwagon in droves! And the last 20% of improvement can often be achieved with conservative whitening, and bonding!

*Adults don't **need** to be treated to prefabricated ideals; they **want** to be treated realistically. With HSB, we can finally deliver, and at the end of the day, they may have a few bucks left over to celebrate their newly found self esteem! - JoAnne G. Rochon, DMD*

FACTOID: A new device is being tested by the FDA which speeds the movement of teeth during most kinds of orthodontic treatment. The device uses vibration energy and may also reduce some of the risks associated with braces (specifically the chance of root damage). Visit the website for further updates.

But I've been told FAST BRACES can hurt Teeth…

As already discussed, but worth repeating, is the latest news to come from an orthodontist's review of the literature. It is that some myths persist about the latest advances in orthodontics which are reducing the speed at which the dental profession is accepting the idea. The actual truth is that faster treatment is safer; that is GREAT news for patients interested in High Speed Braces® or other styles of care that can reduce the time in braces or the number of appointments needed.

Studies prove there is a greater risk of damage to teeth the LONGER braces are worn:

    1. The risk of root damage increases with longer periods of time

in braces. (<u>Most dentists still believe the opposite is true</u>... it was always said in dental school that moving teeth too fast would cause root damage but a study by Dr. Kokich from the University of Seattle has found this to be incorrect, dentists can visit KokichOrthodontics.com for further details).

2. Root damage can range from slight shortening of the roots to severe damage which causes the risk of tooth loss.

3. The risk of cavities or decalcification (spotting damage) increases the longer braces are on as well as for patients with poor brushing and flossing habits.

What can you do if you are already in Braces and think it's taking too long?

If you have been in braces for years and are not making significant improvement or the doctor does not give you any hope, you may want to seek a second opinion. This option will be an added expense, so it may be preferable to discuss your concerns with the doctor, and find out how much more benefit you will get from a longer time in braces.

If the orthodontic provider already has bonded the older style brackets to your teeth, it will not be worth changing to the newer self-ligating style that some believe to be faster or at least capable of reducing the number of appointments- unless you are a complex case at the beginning of your treatment and don't mind paying extra. However, if you are looking for a dental professional to start your treatment, you may want to ask if the brackets they use are the "self-ligating" type (which use clips rather than small elastics to hold the wire in place) because they are at bare minimum easier to clean and allow for shorter office visits. The brand of brackets I recommend may be found on the website and may change as technology advances but each practitioner has his/her biases.

Sadly, there are many examples of situations where someone is in braces much longer than they needed to be. This is sometimes the fault of the practitioner, who may occasionally lose orientation and actually be moving the teeth in the wrong direction. It can also be the patient's fault if they miss appointments or do not follow instructions. Ask to have pictures taken during your treatment, so you can plot your progress and ensure everything is going smoothly towards a better result.

"One of my former assistants was in braces for years longer than she should have been, because her orthodontist was dealing with a difficult personal situation that affected his competence… 'his wacky wife drove him over the edge'. The patient was forced to change orthodontists in the middle of treatment in order to get her braces completed." -mz

What are High Speed Braces® and how do they differ from regular Slow Motion Orthodontics?

Traditional orthodontic philosophy has a similar problem to cosmetic veneer dentistry…the request for ideals can be very costly to patients. In the case of orthodontics it is not money, it is your time. Braces have often taken much more time than necessary as the orthodontists have synthesized very high standards of perfection, which can take years to achieve.

The years of perfecting minor details including midlines of the teeth, and the midlines of the face and the fit of the teeth, are all set out in specific checklists that delay the day the braces can come off. The utopia of perfection, if ever achieved, is carefully photographed and preserved in stone as evidence of a job well done. Then the patient is tossed out into the real world where not everyone flosses or wears their retainer.

In the months following the removal of the braces, the ideals are soon lost as the natural process of settling begins. The bonded wire retainers can lose their grip, and the removable retainers may not be worn nightly or replaced soon enough after they are lost. A small shift can quickly vaporize a year's worth of orthodontic treatment.

Therefore, the premise of High Speed Braces® and other forms of shorter term orthodontics is to make significant improvements in a shorter amount of time, and stress the importance of wearing retainers so the gains are held. This type of treatment combines all the best ideas from both cosmetic dentistry and orthodontics, and uses research on cosmetic perceptions to focus on the most important cosmetic improvements applicable to each patient's situation. The obsessive quest for perfection is substituted with a focus on significant improvement.

We are just happy to make you a little better faster, often for less money than you'd spend on the alternatives.

Not everything can be corrected in a short time, but it is often possible to find a way to reduce the number of appointments and/or the time needed to make a smile look more attractive. "Just Short Of Perfect™" is another brand of treatment style (studied by the author) that recognizes the importance of efficient treatment and the time that can be wasted messing with trying to make things 'perfectio' (whatever that means).

FACTOID: According to some experts, the old style brackets can be made "faster" and allow treatment to be completed in fewer appointments if the wires are "steel tied" into the brackets - rather than being held in with colored elastics. The problem with steel ties is they make wire changes more difficult and make the logical choice of self-ligating brackets (the clip style) worth it. Some brands of clip style brackets have technical problems, so your orthodontic provider hopefully has discovered a brand that has produced excellent results in the past.

Surgical Orthodontic Considerations

The results you get from regular braces and rapid orthodontics can be spectacular,

but orthodontics alone can't always solve all the problems. If a patient has a serious skeletal problem and needs surgical orthodontics, the orthodontist may be able to save time with the use of the faster style brackets called self-ligating brackets (several brands are available) and the most advanced wires available. Another way to speed orthodontic treatment in surgical cases is by having the braces on for as short a time as needed before the surgery. Many times the braces are put on too early, and delays in coordinating the surgery can add years to the time braces are worn. Discussing this before the braces go on is important, due to the damage that can occur from longer times in braces.

So how do you know if you really need surgery? It is a matter of opinion and should not be taken lightly, as *people die every year* from complications. In profile view, if you have a lower jaw that is too big (so your upper front teeth are behind your lower ones) or too small (so your lower teeth bite up into your gums behind your upper front teeth) it may be a sign of a serious skeletal problem. You can also look at yourself in the mirror from the front...if your front teeth show all the way to the gum line even when you're not smiling the bone holding your upper teeth may be too long. Some orthodontists do not feel most skeletal mismatches need to be corrected and instead offer treatment that helps to mask or camouflage the problem; so unless you are handicapped in some way because of a bite problem or serious cosmetic concerns related to this, you may not need it corrected.

FACTOID: The use of TADS or mini-implants in combination with orthodontics has allowed patients to sometimes skip complex and expensive oral surgery procedures. Oral surgeons may be upset, but this is great news for the patients who can be treated with this new technique.

Visit YOUTUBE.com – search terms: High Speed Braces Open Bite

High Speed Braces® vs. Clear Aligners - which are better?

Aligners are clear plastic appliances that slowly move the teeth without the need for braces. Well, that's what the commercials say...in reality there are many conditions that are very difficult to treat with aligners by themselves. When teeth are very crowded and an extraction is needed or the tooth is twisted, an aligner is just not a very efficient way to correct the problem.

Many dentists sign up for aligner programs and do not take other orthodontic training. The aligner company tries to help the dentist work out the best way to use the appliance, and many times the company does not want to admit that another option may be better. Lately, the company has begun to teach ways to do a little pre-straightening with orthodontic brackets and elastics, so the aligner has an easier time. This is better than going for a year or two and finally reverting back to braces, which would have corrected the problem a lot faster from the start.

Aligners work fine for mild orthodontic problems, but for situations that are outside the powers of this appliance, another new development has provided a cutting edge alternative. My experience with aligners is quite limited but the specialists I have studied under tend to prefer the power/speed/control of braces.

The Mini-Breakthrough you've been waiting for... HSB 3 Month Braces™

The development of HSB 3 Month Braces™ came from the High Speed Braces (HSB) Company as a way to give patients interested in porcelain veneers a super-fast alternative to traditional braces. The procedure also competes very well with aligner treatment which costs more and often takes 4-8 times longer.

The procedure typically is only useful in treatment of mild orthodontic problems. The dental professional will analyze your situation and review the issues that can be improved in a short time, and the conditions that will take longer. The training for this unorthodox procedure is outside the traditional programs taught in dental school or orthodontic graduate school: it is looked on with skepticism by those who know little about it. The fact is many recognized leaders of the profession, including some orthodontists, admit that some of the 'old school' techniques, and certainly many of the porcelain makeover programs, do not serve the patients very well. The 3 Month Braces™ program is a form of High Speed Braces®. While most situations cannot be treated this quickly, faster orthodontic treatment is the way of the future.

This new development has been praised by a Harvard-trained orthodontist who lectures and studies developments in orthodontic technology, and uses the exact same brackets recommended for this technique. On the other side, there can be vicious opposition to any new procedure, and some orthodontists have become enraged by the idea of putting a time limit on orthodontic care. It is true that some situations take additional time to correct, but dental professionals need to remember the demands of the clients.

Situations which may be completed in just a few months may include the correction of mild crowding and closing small spaces. It can also be an excellent way to re-treat mild relapses of orthodontic problems, which relate to inadequate retainer usage. In yet another form, HSB 3 Month Braces™ can serve as a 'turbo boost' to an aligner program where the biggest improvements are done with "extreme orthodontics", and then the mild tweaks are completed with removable aligners.

This hybrid of braces and aligners can be a very real answer to the cosmetic demands that people have these days. Given the choice of fast or slow, most people would choose a more rapid correction of a problem. If you've never worn braces, its difficult to understand. While braces of today are much more comfortable than the old style ones of the past, they are still a hassle, and almost everyone asks "when will they come off?"

How can braces do the job so quickly? The dental professionals who use the HSB 3 Month Braces™ technique use the fastest orthodontic technology, alternative goals based on studies of cosmetic perceptions, and simply choose their cases carefully. The "3 month braces" term does not guarantee your teeth will be perfect in exactly three months, the dentist simply anticipates a major cosmetic improvement in a dramatically shorter time than traditional braces or aligners. Some people will be straighter in only weeks, and a few will run overtime, it all depends on the individual situation.

There is a real "sweet spot" at about three months, where suddenly the teeth respond to the technology, and almost overnight they move to a much more attractive position. Many people are simply amazed by the changes that occur in this particular window of time, and while some improvements may still be required, often the primary cosmetic issue is so much better that the patient is ready to get the braces off.

Unless further improvements are required, the patient is scheduled to have the braces removed, and the patient is transitioned into clear retainers or aligners. Generally, aligners are used for last minute minor movements that could not be accomplished with the braces.

An alternative to braces on the outside of the teeth is one that is put on the inside, called "Lingual Braces", and a special bracket has been developed for this purpose which is called MTM (short for Minor Tooth Movement)- or "No Trace™" (as in you can't see them). This technique allows the orthodontist or dentist to treat minor problems in a few months, when significant bite changes are not needed.

Going from braces to retainers in only a few months means having to wear clear retainers at least on a nightly basis, or removable aligners for 24 hours per day (removed only for eating and brushing/flossing). This is not any different from the 'traditional braces patient' that has been in orthodontics for years and years. Teeth just 'have a mind of their own', and you will need to be very faithful to the proper use of the retainers (as discussed earlier).

All too often, people start to neglect the instructions they are given, and their teeth can shift. Very few are lucky enough not to avoid the relapse that occurs when they get sloppy with their retainer program. Signing up for the free service at RetainerReminder.com can help to keep a former ortho patient motivated.

Recent comment made by an Attractive Patient: "If my front teeth overlap again after braces I am just going to get veneers." This tells me a number of things, firstly that patients worry too much about minor details, and secondly they are all too willing to submit themselves to aggressive procedures in an attempt to be perfect. Shorter term orthodontics should be looked upon as a reasonable "touch-up" option which is often a much better choice compared to the alternatives.

Going from Good to Great!

After getting your teeth straightened, you may think that's all that is possible…but it may just be part of what you need to have an attractive smile. Usually, some smile whitening is recommended as a very affordable and safe way to add a little sparkle to your teeth. Not everyone responds the same to 'smile whitening', but almost everyone sees an improvement. Former smokers and coffee drinkers usually are very impressed. While there are many ways to whiten enamel, the tray system and power whitening systems seem to be the most effective. If used properly, 'the take home whitening' can provide similar results to the light-activated power whitening styles …it just takes a little longer due to the lower concentration of peroxide.

Composite bonding may be used to repair minor chips, worn or undersized teeth. A few veneers may sometimes be required, but generally it is best to wait 6-12 months for the teeth to settle in before doing any porcelain work. <u>Note: if you do need veneers after the braces, your teeth will usually need a minimum amount of preparation when compared to "instant orthodontics", where they are basically drilled straight.</u>

As mentioned, gum levels have a huge impact on the look of a smile. Too much gum, or too little, can be an esthetic problem. Sometimes the gums cover too much of the teeth, and need to be repositioned so a nicer amount of tooth is displayed above the gum line. If the gums are a little flabby, the procedure can be done easily by the dentist with a laser or a similar device called a radio-surgery unit. The "gum lift" as it's commonly called, can really give you a much improved finishing touch. Complex gum procedures may be needed if the gum and bone (not just the gums) need to be modified. This often is referred to a periodontist unless the dentist is comfortable performing the procedure. It can takes months to heal from a complex gum lift, so if you still need veneers, waiting months for the gums to recover is usually recommended.

Any missing teeth may be replaced with the treatment that causes the least harm to the remaining ones. Finally, after much effort from you and your dental professionals, your new mouth will look like a million bucks (at a substantial discount, especially if you've used some of the ideas presented in the book).

Classic Car Analogy: Imagine you are buying a vintage car, let's make it a red convertible… one that is going to make you feel like a movie star. You could buy one that's been in a wreck but has been repaired with Bondo® and repainted, it looks very good but you know it's not real. Or you could buy a car that has all the original parts and has been restored by the best in the business; with no expense spared…you simply need to be patient because the owner won't be giving you the keys for a few more years. If you don't quite have the budget for the award winner, you could still look good in the "daily driver" that has been cared for, but is not quite museum material. None of the choices are wrong, but money and time are factors that you have control over and may factor in your decision. Dental work is a little like that.

Retainers and the Secret to keeping your Teeth Straight

Retainers are dental appliances that are used to keep teeth in a particular position - usually after they have been moved with some type of orthodontic procedure. There are a number of retainers to choose from, and some are removable and others are not. <u>The current research suggests that the key to keeping your teeth straight after braces is not how long you wear the braces, it's how long you wear your retainers.</u>

The bonded retainers are typically a fitted wire that is glued to the inside of the teeth. It is hidden from sight, and soon it is not even noticeable to your tongue. They are used to keep the lower front teeth straight. Bonded wires can make flossing difficult, and more frequent cleanings are needed. The lingual wire retainer does loosen and fall off fairly commonly.

The Bottom Line

There are thousands of outstanding cosmetic dentists, orthodontists and other dental professionals in North America. Even the best practitioners experience a certain number of failures, but that is not my concern. The best dental care can be destroyed by patient neglect, wear and tear, and exposure to the harsh environment of the mouth - that's simply good for business. The problem is that many dental professionals are still caught in the 90's style of cosmetic treatment, or do not want to respond to the demands people have. There may only be a couple of 'Veneer Nazis' in every major city, but they will soon become extinct.

The *New Age* cosmetic dentist will know when to use porcelain veneers and when to use other means to make your smile look better. Porcelain veneers are not dangerous if used properly, but advances have made alternatives a better choice in many situations. Orthodontists will use more efficient techniques and compete with former cosmetic dentists for patients wanting shorter treatment times in braces (without headgear or barbaric appliances like the Herbst).

It may take a number of years for cosmetic dentists to retrain and learn to use the latest developments, which allow for significant aesthetic improvements without resorting to reckless drilling of teeth. Similarly, the orthodontic practitioners will feel the pressure to reduce their treatment times, and learn different skills to compete with innovations, in the ever-changing marketplace. *Not every situation can or should be treated with the new styles of care shared in this book, but it is important to know there are alternatives you may not be told about without specifically asking.* I hope you will find a dental team who understands the importance of giving you as many conservative and affordable options as possible, before you make your decision to change your smile. There are dental professionals that are learning more about these innovations so do your homework.

There was simply no way we could pack everything we wanted to share in this book, so I hope you will continue to uncover even more insider secrets by staying in touch. PLEASE continue to see your dental team regularly to keep your dental health at its optimum level. Finally **DO NOT EVEN THINK about getting a smile makeover unless you have read this book from cover to cover, visited the website, and discussed some of the controversial suggestions with your most trusted dental advisors.**

If you have a complex situation, seek opinions from a general dentist, a cosmetic dentist who has taken some orthodontic courses in addition to the veneer programs, a friendly orthodontist and even a prosthodontist (if an extreme makeover has been recommended) to help find the most appropriate treatment for your individual situation. It's better to spend a thousand in consultation fees to find out about a safer alternative than wasting ten or twenty times that amount and jumping into something from which there is no going back.

Thanks for reading this book. If you would like to join me in making an additional donation to SmileTrain.org, some of the money you saved from not doing an *extreme smile makeover* will make a child with cleft lip/palate very happy. In spite of all my babbling, Smiles are important.

THANKS to those who have contributed!

I would like to thank my late father who gave me the inspiration to expose wrongdoings. I grew up with significant political and religious exposure, where others were constantly threatening our livelihood, creating negative publicity, scandal and controversy. This created a need to be an antiestablishmentarian (… I've only typed it once in my life). Thanks to my mother for inspiring creativity and alternative beliefs. My family has put up with hundreds of lost hours due to my work schedule, and my never-ending project development.

I express my gratitude to my staff and colleagues with whom I have worked and studied. Many thanks to my mentors and patients who helped me learn to fix teeth a little better than when I escaped from dental school. Thanks to Geoff Nanton for hours of frustration editing my rantings. Thanks for legal advice from the Law Offices of Karen J. Bernstein LLC, New York City and Nick Nanton of Dicks & Nanton. I appreciate the input from the guest critics, even though some disagreed with some of my advice. Finally, thank you to the select group of dental professionals who tried to stop me from doing what I thought was right…you inspired me even more than you can imagine!

The opinions in this book are based on the most recent research reviewed by the author and are not presented to provide individual advice. You are encouraged to consult with a trusted dental professional for interpretation of how this information may affect your treatment. Use of information in this book is at your own risk and no liability is assumed by the author or any disseminator of this information for any damage whatsoever that occurs from use of information in this publication or on the websites. Some of the information is provided for entertainment value, and may in fact not be funny to all readers. Some information may be inaccurate or affected by the biases of the author. Omissions and errors are included in the price of the book and if possible they may be corrected on the website. Trade names and marks belong to the respective companies mentioned and are not implied to belong to the author. All corporate names, trademarks, and institutional affiliations are for identification purposes only, and do not constitute any form of approval or endorsement of this book. Dr. Zuk provides consulting services to dentists, orthodontists and a number of the companies mentioned in this publication. Correspondence may be directed through the website ConfessionsofaFormerCosmeticDentist.com.

Copyright 2009 Dr. M.Y. Zuk

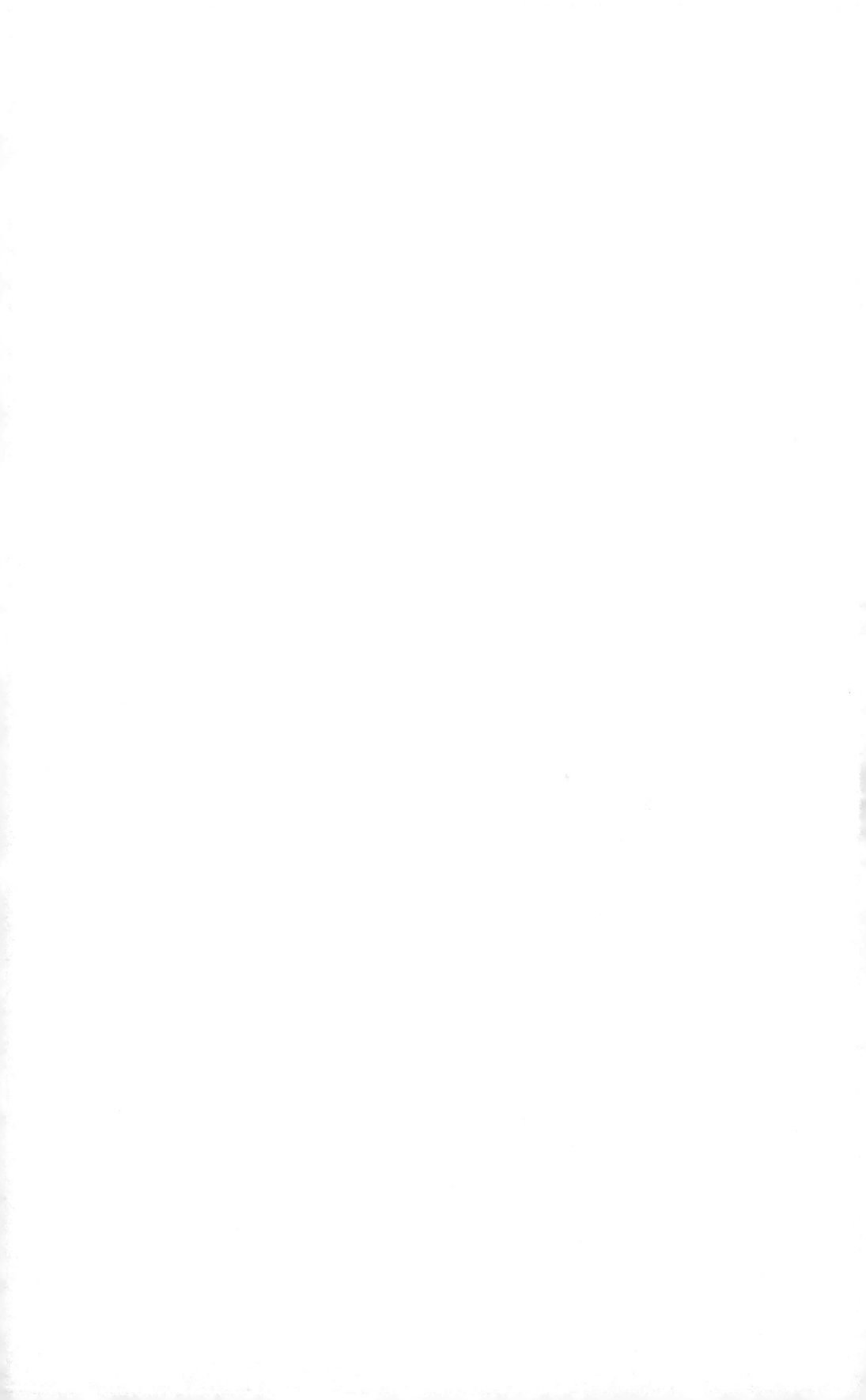

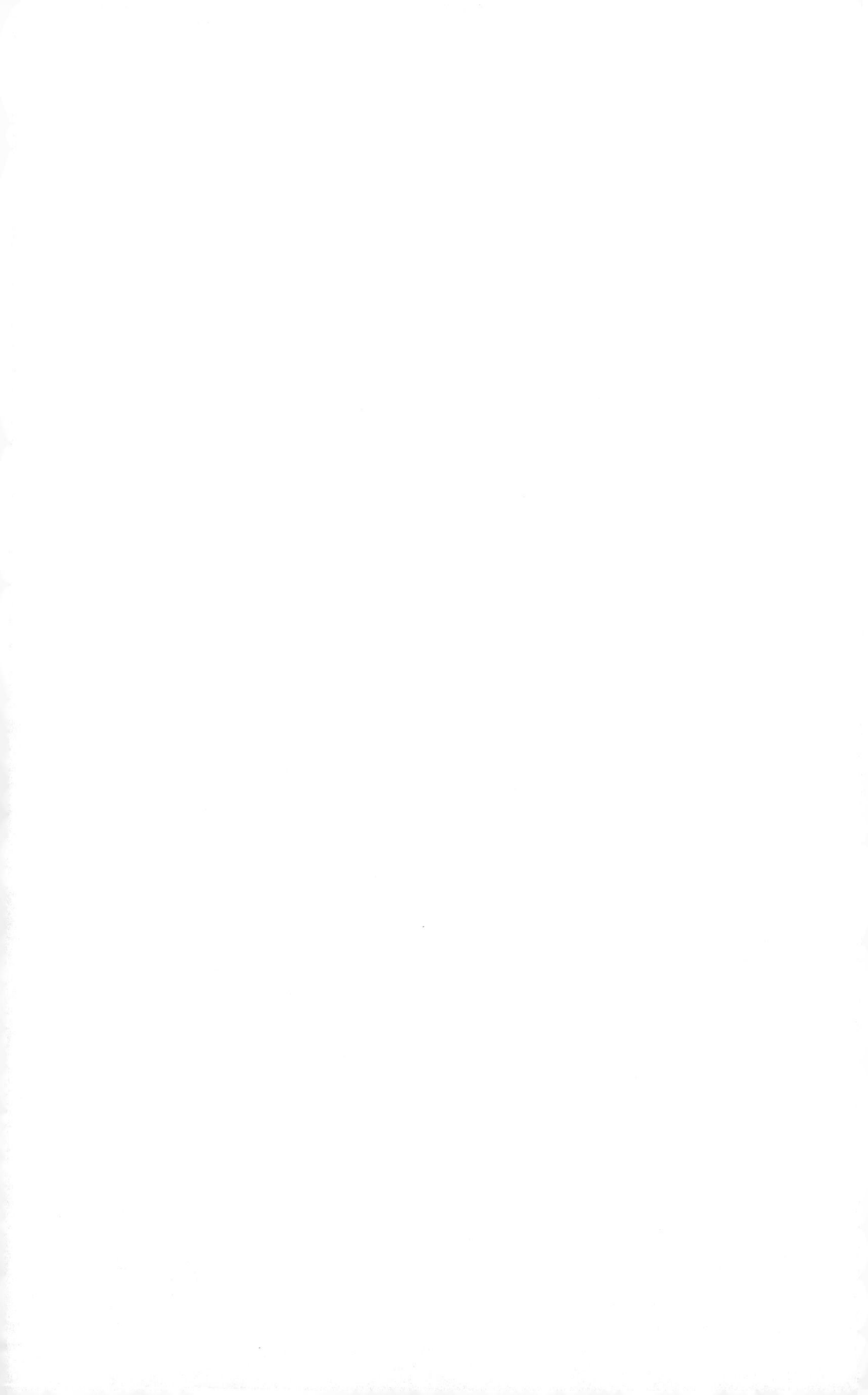